ASHLEY BROWN'S

what to eat

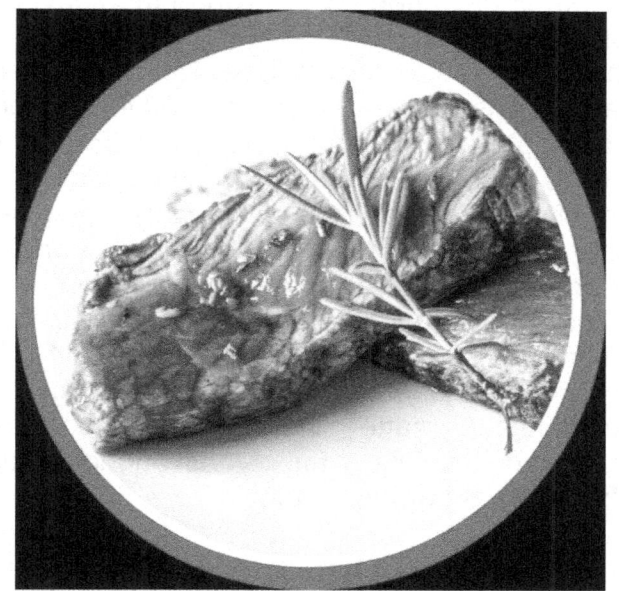

to get fit

A COMPLETE GUIDE TO THE KETOGENIC DIET

4 WEEKS OF MEAL PLANNING + SHOPPING LISTS

120 EASY AND TASTY RECIPES

30 DESSERT RECIPES INCLUDED

All Rights Reserved. No part of this publication or the information in it may be quoted from or reproduced in any form by means such as printing, scanning, photocopying or otherwise without prior written permission of the copyright holder.

Declaimer and Terms of Use: Effort has been made to ensure that the information in this book is accurate and complete, however, the author and the publisher do not warrant the accuracy of the information, text and graphics contained within the book due to the rapidly changing nature of science, research, known and unknown facts and internet. The author and the publisher do not hold any responsibility for errors, omissions or contrary interpretation of the subject matter herein. This book is presented solely for motivational and informational purposes only.

Contents

Introduction **9**
Chapter 1: What is the Ketogenic Diet? **11**

Types of Ketogenic Diet 14
Standard Ketogenic Diet 14
Cyclical Ketogenic Diet 15
Targeted Ketogenic Diet 16

Chapter 2: What to Know **17**

Having the Right Mindset 17
Preparing Your Kitchen 18
Be Prepared for Those First Weeks 19
The Keto Flu 19
Controlling Those Sugar Cravings 20

Chapter 3: Benefits of the Ketogenic Diet **21**

Weight loss 21
Improved mental focus 21
Treatment for Type 2 Diabetes 23
Not a Zero-Carb Diet 23
Ketogenic Diets Help with Epilepsy 23
Ketogenic Diets Help Fight Many Diseases 24
You will be more energised 25
Improved Digestion 26

Chapter 4: How to Start **28**

What You Should Eat 28
Do Not Eat 37

Chapter 5: Dangers and Side Effects of the Ketogenic Diet and How to Avoid Them **39**

Keto Flu 39
Bad Breath 39
Leg cramps 41
Keto Rash 43

Drawbacks 46
Effects of the Ketogenic Diet 46
Chapter 6: How to Attain Ketosis 53

Breathalyzer 54
Pee Ketone Strips 54
Perception 54
Chapter 7: Useful Tips 55

Reading Nutrition Labels 55
Sleeping During Ketosis 56
Ketogenic Diet and Stress 56
Chapter 8: Breakfast Recipes 59

1. Avocado Stuffed with Tuna 60
2. Tuna in Cucumber 61
3. Small Keto Pies 62
4. Keto Wraps 64
5. Chicken Omelet 66
6. Eggs in Pepper 68
7. Naan Bread and Butter 70
8. Breakfast Tuna Salad 72
9. Deviled Eggs 73
10. Low-Carb Muffins with Whey 74
11. Spinach Rolls 75
12. Breakfast Smoothie 77
13. Low-Carb Breakfast Balls 78
14. Keto Muffins with Chicken 79
15. Borecole with Curry 80
16. Eggs on Sour Cream 81
17. Low-Carb Bacon Muffins 82
18. Zucchini in Yogurt 83
19. Gluten-Free, Keto Coconut Bread 84
20. Baked Brussels Sprout with Garlic 85
21. Ketogenic Protein Muffins 86
22. Fried Peppers with Cauliflowers 87

23. Eggs Sauce 89
24. Keto Breakfast 90
25. Bacon Burger 92
26. Pesto Scrambled Eggs 94
27. Keto Waffles with Pumpkin Spice 95
28. Keto Cheese Tacos 97
29. Chive and Bacon Omelet 101
30. Baked Avocados with Eggs and Bacon 103

Chapter 9: Lunch Recipes 105

31. Beef Burritos 106
32. Open-Faced Prosciutto and Sandwich 108
33. The Keto Cubano 110
34. Keto Monkey Bread 112
35. Beef Stew 114
36. Beef Welly 115
37. Salmon Fish Cakes 117
38. Bistro Steak Salad with Horseradish Dressing .. 119
39. Low-Carb Mayonnaise for the Dressing 121
40. Caprese Salad 122
41. Egg Salad Stuffed Avocado 124
42. Thai Pork Salad 126
43. Vegetarian Club Salad 128
44. Cumin Spiced Beef Wraps 130
45. Balsamic Beef Pot Roast 132
46. Cheeseburger Calzone 134
47. Vegetarian Keto Burger on a Bun 136
48. Barbecue Pulled Chicken in the Slow Cooker 138
49. Beef Patties 140
50. Ground Beef Bacon Cheeseburger 142
51. BBQ & Bacon Cheeseburger Waffles 144
52. Thai Beef 146
54. Portobello Bun Cheeseburgers 149
55. BBQ Pulled Beef Sando – Slow Cooker 151

56. Bone Broth for the BBQ 153
57. Beef Wellington 154
58. Mississippi Chuck Roast 156
59. Nacho Steak – Skillet Style 158
60. Steak-Lovers Slow-Cooked Chili 160

Chapter 10: Dinner Recipes 162

61. Chicken and Asparagus Pan Dinner 163
62. Chicken Kiev 165
63. Chicken Pad Thai 167
64. Chicken Parmesan 169
65. Chicken Smothered in Creamy Sauce 171
66. Chicken Stuffed Avocado—Cajun Style 173
67. Coconut Curry Chicken Tenders 175
68. Beef Pot Roast 177
69. Italian Chicken and Cauliflower Casserole 178
70. Italian Chicken & Egg Bake 180
71. Kung Pao Chicken 182
72. Nacho Chicken Casserole 184
73. Tikka Masala Chicken – Slow Cooker 186
74. Pizza Goodies BBQ Meat-Lover's Pizza 188
75. Beefy Pizza 190
76. Chicken Fried Pork Chops 191
77. Parmesan Crusted Pork Chops 193
78. Skillet Style Sausage and Cabbage Melt 195
79. Squash and Sausage Casserole 197
80. Chili Lime Cod 199
81. Pan Fried Cod 201
82. Grilled Salmon 203
83. Sushi 205
84. Walnut Crusted Salmon 207
85. One-Pot Shrimp Alfredo 209
86. Loaded Tuna Fish Salad 211
87. Tuna Tartare 212

88. Chipotle Fish Tacos 214
89. Bell Pepper Basil Pizza 216

Chapter 11: Desserts 219

90. Cheesy Brussels Sprouts 220
91. Mini Chocolate Cakes 221
92. Poached Eggs 222
93. Ricotta Lemon Cheesecake 223
94. Wheat Belly Yogurt 225
95. Eggs in a Cup 226
96. Vanilla Bean Cheesecake 228
97. Greek Yogurt 229
98. Garlic Spread 231
99. Peanut Butter Cheesecake 232
100. Pumpkin Pecan Cake 233
101. Chocolate Cream 235
102. Butter Pancakes 237
103. Raspberry Cookies 239
104. Vanilla Mousse with Chocolate Sauce 241
105. Sweet Almond Buns 243
106. Cocoa Patties 245
107. Easy Almond Bars 246
108. Pumpkin Pie Pancakes 248
109. Coconut Brownies with Raspberries 250
110. Chocolate Chip Cookies 252
111. Vanilla Cream 254
112. Cheesecake with Warm Chocolate Sauce 256
113. Peanut Butter Brownies 258
114. Chocolate Chip Keto Brownies 260
115. Raspberry Yogurt with Avocado 262
116. Cherry Pudding 264
117. Creamy Raspberry Cake 266
118. Strawberry Chocolate Fudge 268
119. Apple Lemon Pie 270

120. Almond Strawberry Squares..................................272
Chapter 12: 4 Weeks of Meal Planning 274
Week 1: Shopping List..274
Week 2: Shopping List..277
Week 3: Shopping list 279
Week 4: Shopping List..282
Chapter 13: Volume conversion tables.......... 284
Conclusion 287

Introduction

Dear Reader,

First of all, I would like to thank you for buying this book and wish you good luck during your tasty diet!

The following chapters will provide you 120 recipes, and information on the benefits of the Ketogenic Diet.

Finding healthy and easy recipes is one of the biggest challenges you'll face when on a Ketogenic Diet. In our modern lives, we rarely have time to cook for ourselves every single day. Between work, bringing kids to practice and cleaning up around the house, cooking healthy meals is usually the first thing to suffer.

All the recipes here take less than an hour of prep time. However, most recipes take only 15 minutes, or less, to make. Once the initial prep work is done, it's just a matter of set it and forget it. Then, when you come home, you have a delicious Ketogenic meal to enjoy with your family!

The book is designed to make finding the perfect recipe easy. The book is divided into 4 parts: breakfast, lunch, dinner and desserts. Under each section, recipes are organized from the quickest total time to make, to the longest. Each recipe includes full nutritional information, so there's no guessing how many carbs you're eating. Enjoy!

Sincerely yours,
Ashley Brown

Chapter 1: What is the Ketogenic Diet?

Ketogenic dieters consume fewer calories and focus on high-fat, low-carb options, using food that offers some medical advantages, including weight reduction. For a long time, individuals suspected that fat influenced them to gain fat; subsequently, this prompted many people endeavoring to get more fit by lessening their significant admission by taking low-fat substitutes of various sustenances. Because of the enormous rush of significant influences you to fat, distinctive subsistence producers needed to make a move to enable individuals to quit getting fat. They did so by lessening the measure of fat in different nourishment. There was an issue with sustenance not being great because of decreased fat levels, so these organizations needed to search for ways to make low-fat nourishment desirable. Here is the thing that they did. To make low-fat food still taste great, they included more sugar. Lamentably, rather than individuals shedding pounds, they put on weight. At that point you may ask: Why is that so?

In the current past, there have been more examinations taking a gander at whether heavy influences you to fat and the conclusion is that sugar is the thing that changes you to fat. How is that so? When you abstain from high-carb food, the pancreas discharges insulin to make the glucose accessible to platelets and to oversee glucose levels. Insulin encourages the cells to ingest glucose from the circulatory system, and, without it (insulin), the cells would keep from glucose, regardless of the possibility that the circulatory system has an abundance of glucose! The body cells ingest some glucose for use in metabolic exercises, with the overabundance glucose being changed over to fat for capacity. Understand that the body's essential wellspring of fuel is glucose and, as long as the body has an adequate supply of glucose, it won't consume fat.

The Ketogenic eat in a way that puts the body in a state where it consumes fat for vitality (ketosis). When you take on a low-card eating regimen with sufficient protein and high in fat, the level of glucose (the body's essential wellspring of fuel) is small; consequently, the body is compelled to search for different wellsprings of fuel; subsequently swinging to fats. Hence, ketosis is a metabolic state where lipids are separated in the liver into ketones for vitality. We will take a more detailed gander at ketosis in substantially in a later section. For the present, let us attempt to comprehend how abstaining from certain foods works and has helped many individuals get in shape.

Why the Ketogenic Diet Is Effective for Weight Loss

1: According to many individuals, a couple of days after pulling back from starches, they encountered expanded vitality levels. This is because a gram of fat has abundant dietary energy. When you feel more energetic, you are more likely to take part in various activities, including working out to consume fat. Likewise, once you begin exploring a significantly improved lifestyle, you are probably not going to surrender to enthusiastic eating, which is the principal offender for some individuals who are overweight.

2: The ketogenic slim down works since it is satisfying. As previously said, a ketogenic calorie count is high in fat, adequate protein and low-carb. Fats are satisfying, as are proteins. In this way, you will feel full for longer and have no compelling reason to indulge.

3: The Ketogenic consume fewer calories, which enacts fat digestion

on account of the decreased level of insulin in the body. Given that you decline your admission of carbs, your blood has less of glucose, which implies that there won't be a requirement for the discharge of high measures of insulin. Remember that other than encouraging the cells to ingest glucose, insulin has the impact of repressing fat digestion (lipolysis). Preferably, it advances fat stockpiling and glycogen collection (glycolysis). With decreased insulin levels, your body can adequately begin utilizing fats since there is no hindrance.

With that comprehension of how the ketogenic count calories, let us now look at what happens to your body when on a ketogenic diet, consuming fewer calories.

Types of Ketogenic Diet

Now that you're considering bringing the Ketogenic Diet into your wellness routine, you need to decide which version of the Ketogenic diet is the right one for you. There are three versions: Standard Ketogenic Diet, Cyclical Ketogenic Diet, and Targeted Ketogenic Diet.

Why three? The Ketogenic Diet that is right for you depends on your level of fitness and level of exercise intensity each week. For most individuals, the standard Ketogenic food should be the right fit. However, if you are a high-intensity athlete, a bodybuilder, marathoner or something similar, then you might want to consider cyclical or targeted Keto. Let's go over exactly what these three Ketogenic Diets involve.

Standard Ketogenic Diet
The Standard Ketogenic Diet is, basically, the one we've been talking about this whole time. This food is best for people who have low, moderate or moderately high levels of physical activity, and who need to lose weight. If you fit into this category, try using the Standard

Ketogenic Diet before you check out the other two.

In the Standard Ketogenic diet, you follow the prescribed amounts of fats, carbs and protein: 80% fat, 15% protein, and 5% carbs. As long as you feel like you have energy, and you aren't trying to train for a marathon or compete in Olympic-level sports, this diet should be sufficient to give you energy while promoting weight loss.

Cyclical Ketogenic Diet

In this version, athletes can have a day of carb bulking before engaging in intense athletic activity. This food is only for athletes or bodybuilders who are very advanced in their workout regimen. The goal of this style of Keto is to completely deplete the glycogen stored in your muscles in between workouts.

When practicing the Cyclical Ketogenic Diet, you'll continue to follow the high-fat, shallow carb model for most of your time. However, occasionally, once a week or for two days during the week, you can eat medium to high carbs. It allows your muscles to store up to glycogen, which will give you a boost of energy throughout the week. If you do not need weight loss, you can have two high-carb days, and two medium-carb days during the week, with the remaining three days being high-fat.

Targeted Ketogenic Diet

In the Targeted Ketogenic Diet version of the menu, carb bulking is used just before exercise to provide a sudden boost of energy. The goal of targeted Keto is to maintain the glycogen stores in the muscles. Again, this version of the Ketogenic diet is only for elite athletes.

If you're a high-intensity athlete, working out four or five days each week, you can use targeted Keto to give your muscles a boost before or after each workout. It can help prevent the fatigue or lack of muscle gain that is sometimes attributed to the Standard Ketogenic Diet.

How does this work? Targeted Keto works by allowing you to eat a high-carb meal about two hours before your next intense workout, and within one hour after the workout. How many carbs you eat depends on your body, diet and energy level. It may take some time to figure out what is right for you.

Chapter 2: What to Know Before You Start Your Keto Journey

Getting ready to go Keto may seem like an intimidating task, but, with the right preparation, it doesn't need to be. The Ketogenic Diet is a significant change from the standard American diet, but if you come into it with the right tools and the right mentality, you will be astounded by what you can achieve.

Having the Right Mindset

One of the best things you can do is switch your thinking from long-term to short-term. Of course, you have long-term goals, but if you only focus on the long-term, things can feel overwhelming. Instead, try setting more immediate short-term aims to help you get through the transition period.

Commit to follow a strict Ketogenic Diet for just one month before you take your first cheat day. If you can stick to thinking responsibly, you will be Keto-adapted and will see the beginning of your incredible results.

The other aspect of your mind that you need to be ready for is cravings. Cravings are a healthy and natural part of every diet. At some point during that first month, you will feel cravings for carbs.

There are two things you can do to overcome these desires. The first is to remind yourself that cravings will get less intense over time. If you can commit to that first month, you will feel your needs decrease significantly.

Preparing Your Kitchen

Another essential step in going Keto is getting your kitchen in order. If you try to be on the Ketogenic Diet, but your kitchen is full of bread, pasta, and processed foods, you're going to give in to your cravings immediately. Once you've decided to commit to the Ketogenic Diet, you should take a few days to prepare your kitchen. Get rid of craving foods, processed foods and all the foods that don't fit into the Ketogenic Diet.

If you've got a family to feed, and they aren't going to be Keto, consider making a cabinet that is just for your Ketogenic foods. Separate out the non-Ketogenic diets that could trigger cravings, and promise yourself not to look in those drawers or cabinets.

So, what food should you have in your kitchen?

At least at the beginning of your Ketogenic journey, make sure to keep it simple. Don't try to make fancy, grain-free Keto bread or crackers, and stay away from Keto desserts. Fill your refrigerator with vegetables and Keto-approved cheeses. Buy a few different types of meat and plenty of eggs. Learn how to make three or four quick and easy Keto meals, such as the ones found in the meal plan at the end of this book, and mentally prepare yourself to eat those during the first weeks.

Be Prepared for Those First Weeks

The first days and weeks of the Ketogenic Diet are some of the hardest that you'll go through. That's why taking steps to prepare your mindset and supply your kitchen are so important. If you have the right tools in place, you'll be able to get through those first difficult days. During the first weeks of Keto, your body and mind will go through many changes. You'll lose weight, but then plateau. You'll feel angry, hungry, tired and frustrated.

The Keto Flu

The Keto Flu is a nickname for the physical changes that your body goes through when you first give up on carbohydrates. Because you're going without carbohydrates probably for the first time, your body might react poorly. Common symptoms of the Keto Flu are headaches, nausea, fatigue and other uncomfortable physical reactions.

As a caveat, not everyone experiences the Keto Flu, and there are varying degrees of intensity. You might find your head in a fog for a few days. You may feel tired, or you may become incredibly sick. Gradually reduce your carbohydrate consumption over 4 to 6 weeks before switching entirely to Keto. It can prevent the extreme symptoms of the Keto Flu. Once the Keto Flu symptoms start to hit, the best thing you can do is increase your salt and fluid intake by drinking cups of bouillon.

Most of all, if you feel yourself getting sick and uncomfortable during the first weeks of Keto, don't panic! Know that this is normal, and if you want support to get through it, there are plenty of online communities full of people who want to help you get the most out of Keto.

Controlling Those Sugar Cravings

No doubt about it, you will be plagued by cravings for sugar during those first few weeks on Keto. Especially when you get hungry or need a snack, the desire to eat some bread, cake or cookies will be high. Luckily, there are ways to beat these cravings. The best way to overcome cravings is being prepared. Pay attention to your body's cycles. What time do you usually get hungry?

Some high-fat, Keto-approved snacks to carry around with you are natural, low-carb peanut butter with carrots, unprocessed cheeses or dark chocolate. Having those on hand will prevent you from heading to the nearest vending machine and ruining your diet.

Initial Weight Loss

Most people experience a drop in their body weight after the first week of Keto. While, of course, this is exciting and motivating, you should also know that this was mostly water weight and excess carbohydrate stored in your body. You may experience a plateau, or slower weight loss, afterward. Don't be bummed out. If you stick with the Ketogenic Diet, the pounds will melt away. Commit to 30, then 60, and then 90 days and watch your body transform.

Chapter 3: Benefits of the Ketogenic Diet

Proper planning is essential in starting a Keto Diet. It means that you will have to come up with a viable diet plan to stick to. How fast you will reach a ketogenic state depends on the foods that will compose your menu, as well as some foods that you eat. Remember the fewer carbohydrates you take, the faster you will enter ketosis.

The Keto Diet offers a ton of benefits from weight loss to improving mental focus and physical performance, among others.

Weight loss

Weight loss is a common effect of a Ketogenic Diet. When a person reaches the state of ketosis, the body burns fat in the liver and produces ketones. It turns the body into an active and efficient fat burning machine, where it taps and burns its fat reserves to generate ketones as fuel for the organization.

Improved mental focus

Increased focus and concentration is one of the standard effects of a ketone diet. When you reach the state of ketosis, the brain receives and uses a constant flow of ketones. In fact, many people, even those who are already physically fit, still rely on the ketone diet to improve their mental performance. Moreover, this diet avoids dramatic fluctuations in blood sugar levels.

Interestingly, many people still think that proper brain functions require lots of carbohydrates. However, this is only true if ketones are not available.

After about a week of adapting to a Ketogenic Diet, the brain and the body can function smoothly on ketones. However, it is worth noting that before you reach this stage, you will first have to face the everyday challenges that accompany most low-carb diets, such as a headache, mood swings and difficulty in concentrating. Once you pass the initial stages of hardship, you can enjoy higher energy levels, as well as better mental focus.

Increased Physical Endurance

Since a ketone diet will allow you to have access to all the energy of your fat reserves, it can significantly develop your physical endurance.

The body's storage of carbohydrates (glycogen) can only last for a few hours of physical activity, even less. But, your fat reserves have enough energy to last for weeks, even months.

Since most people these days are used to tapping their storage of carbohydrates as a source of energy, their fat reserves are not readily available, not even to fuel their brain. It results in needing to eat before, during and after a workout, or also just to avoid hunger and fuel your day-to-day activities. The Ketogenic Diet solves this problem by allowing you to tap your fat reserves to feed not only your body, but also your brain. And, unlike other foods that are just good for a month or two, the state of ketosis can last forever.

Treatment for Type 2 Diabetes

Since the ketone diet is a low-carb diet, it is proven to be effective in reversing Type 2 Diabetes. The primary cause of Type 2 Diabetes is high blood sugar. Since this sugar comes from the carbs that you eat, it means that the less sugar you eat, the less sugar will be present in the blood which, in turn, will lower your blood sugar level. A dramatic drop in blood sugar level is a natural part of the ketone diet. Always keep in mind that if you are already taking medications for Type 2 Diabetes, you will have to adjust the dosage once you engage in a ketone diet to avoid your blood sugar from dropping too low. It is also an excellent way to control Type 1 Diabetes.

Not a Zero-Carb Diet

A ketone diet does not ultimately remove all carbohydrates from your diet. It merely imposes a limitation or restriction on some carbs that you eat. Your carbs should come from nuts, vegetables and dairy products. You must avoid eating any refined carbohydrates, such as starch (beans, potatoes and legumes), wheat (bread, cereals, pasta), and fruits. Exceptions to these are berries, avocado and star fruits, which can be taken in moderation.

Ketogenic Diets Help with Epilepsy

This is returning to the literal roots of the initial usage of the Ketogenic Diet. Since the time of the ancients, the prescribed treatment for fits, which we now know as epileptic seizures, was to allow the patient to go on a fast or for the patients to not consume sugar or starches. Now we know of course that this route would set the body down the path of being converted to a fat burner, and thereby produce ketones, which is the key ingredient for the effective treatment of Epilepsy.

Documented usage began from the early-1900s where it was used as a go-to approach for epileptic seizures. You would have gathered from the early parts of this book that this form of treatment progressed well into the 1940s, where the inventions of anti-epileptic medicines, which offered fast relief of the symptoms, put this natural dietary approach on the backburner.

Fortunately, the diet rediscovered some of its past popularity when Hollywood made a movie about it and, right now, we have a healthy wave of adopters who are enjoying epilepsy-free lives without the side effects of medications. This proves that good things do last, yes sometimes they get buried and lost perhaps, but ultimately it will always come back if we look hard enough.

Ketogenic Diets Help Fight Many Diseases

Ketogenic Diets are known to have the potential to fight diseases such as Polycystic Ovary Syndrome (PCOS), Alzheimer's, depression, traumatic brain injury, stroke and others that plague our present generations. There are many studies conducted by reputable institutions that have shown multiple promising results in this aspect. Cancer has also been one of the diseases which is receiving notice with regards to the Ketogenic Diet, as indicated in growing research on "starving" cancer cells.

The notion of starving cancer cells is not new. It was first brought up back in 1924 by German scientist Otto Warburg who proposed that the prime cause of cancer was derived from the fermentation of sugar within the body's cells. The primary notion is to remove the sugar or glucose consumption, replace it with dietary fat and the cancer cells, starved of its usual fuel, will then die. It is this book's hope that more clinical trials and research can be done to further this hypothesis. Who knows, we might just have a powerful deterrent for cancer.

You will be more energised

Ketones are a more reliable and sustaining source of energy, and you will feel this energy surging through your body. Chronic fatigue symptoms that you had been experiencing up until now will go away, and you will feel more energetic when you introduce Keto Diets into your lifestyle.

Because of the cut in reliance on energy from carbs, your body will be spared the "sugar rush" effect, where you get brief surges of energy followed by periods of fatigue. With ketones as your main energy source, your body will constantly be fueled due to the ever-present fat burning process going on, just like a light bulb that remains lit consistently, without flickers and intermittent outages.

Your Mood is Enhanced, and There is Increased Clarity in Thought

Both of these improvements are credited to ketone bodies that are beneficial in stabilising and controlling neurotransmitters, such as dopamine and serotonin. The stabilisation of these neurotransmitters helps you control your moods better and improve the clarity of thought.

Doctors who have tracked many of their patients on Keto Diets say that they have seen improved cognitive functions as well as reduced anxiety. The patients also tend to have better memory and seem to be able to enjoy and live life with lesser dependency on drugs and medications.

Improved Digestion

By shifting to a Keto Diet and reducing sugar and carb intake, you will experience improved digestion and your gut health will also see significant improvement. This is also associated with reduced sugar and grain consumption. The usual bloating and feelings of indigestion will tend to subside.

Enjoy Better Sleep

With the adoption of the Ketogenic Diet, you will be more inclined to enjoy a good night's rest. Many Keto-adapted practitioners report that after being in ketosis, they can sleep throughout the night like a baby, without sleep being interrupted in fits and being started awake. These improvements are linked to reduced glucose intake in the daily diet, which tends to facilitate a lower level of chronic inflammation in the system, thereby allowing the body to ease itself and remain easily in deeper rest.

Chapter 4: How to Start and What You Can Eat

What You Should Eat

Not in any way like fasting, the Ketogenic thin down urges you to eat. Regardless, you can't just eat any sustenance. In a keto diet, you should merely eat foods that are low in carbs, attractive in protein and high in fats.

Meats

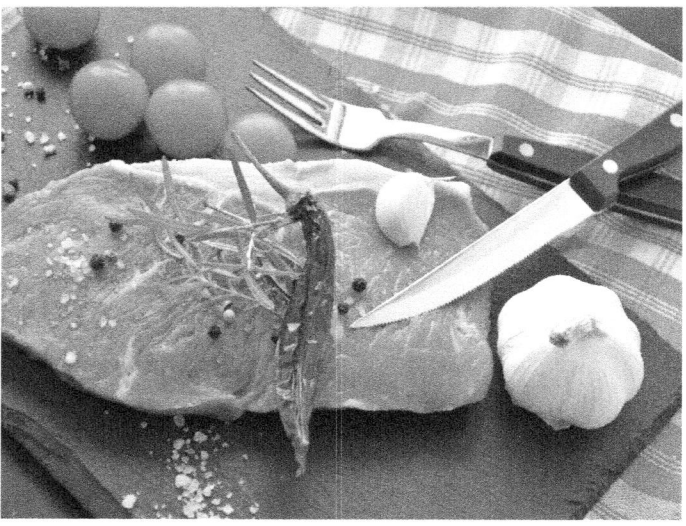

Stick to meats that have an ideal measure of protein and low-carb substance, such as ground sirloin sandwich, point, eggs, etc. Eat wild and avoid developed fish.

Vegetables

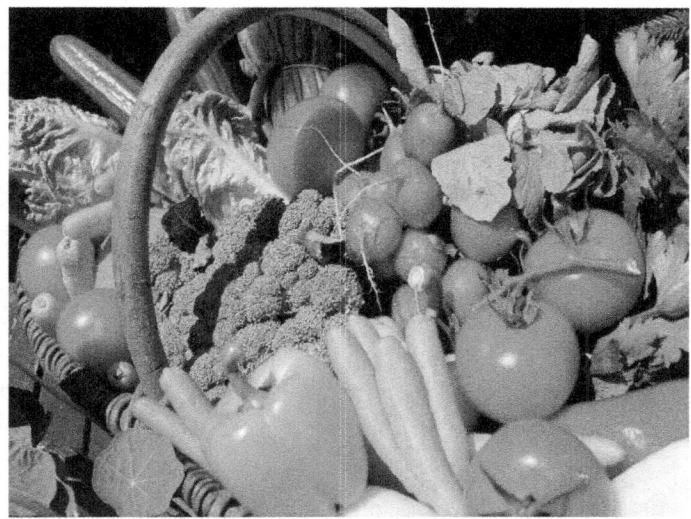

Eat verdant greens like turnips, collards, spinach and kale. You can also eat over the ground vegetables, such as broccoli, squash, cauliflower and zucchini.

High-Fat Dairy

High-fat sustenance's are a standard bit of a Keto Fiet. Fat impacts you to feel full for a more expanded period. Delineations: high fat cream, margarine, and unusual cheeses.

Nuts and Seeds

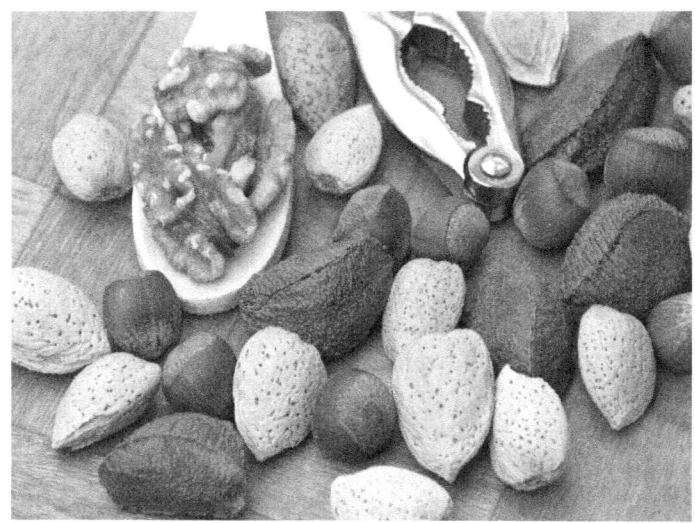

Nuts and seeds are squeezed with supplements that can empower your body to stay thin and sound. Try options such as macadamias, almonds, walnuts and sunflower seeds.

Berries

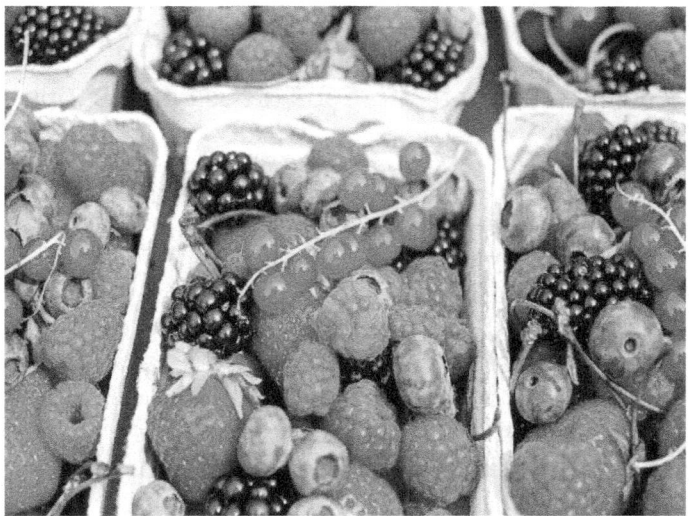

Sweeteners

Use sweeteners that have the most negligible count of sugars, such as Splenda, Stevia, cleric essential items, Sweet 'n' Low, etc.

Distinctive Fats

Other incredible wellsprings of fats that you can unite into your keto diet are high-fat servings of blended greens dressing, coconut oil and drenched fats.

Keep in mind that a typical ketone eating regimen typically follows a 70% Fats, 25% Protein and 5% Carbohydrates plan.

It is proposed to take between 20-30g of net carbs consistently to expend fewer calories. Regardless, if you have to hit ketosis quickly, you may consider fewer carbs and keep your glucose levels low. In case getting more fit is your inspiration of doing a keto diet, it is decidedly recommended that you watch your total sugars and net starches. When you participate in a ketone eating routine and get yourself hungry, you can check your yearning by eating nuts, nutty spread, cheddar and seeds.

Broccoli

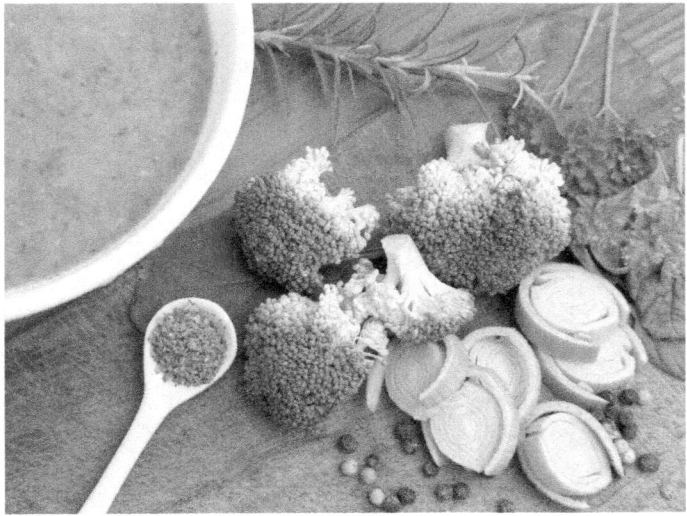

Broccoli is outstandingly regular on a ketone diet. It is loaded with Vitamins C and K. More importantly, a measure of broccoli just contains 4g net carbs. Distinctive examinations show that the people who have Type 2 Diabetes can benefit from eating broccoli, since it cuts down insulin resistance. Broccoli can shield you from a couple of types of development. It is thought of as a staple in a Keto Diet.

Asparagus

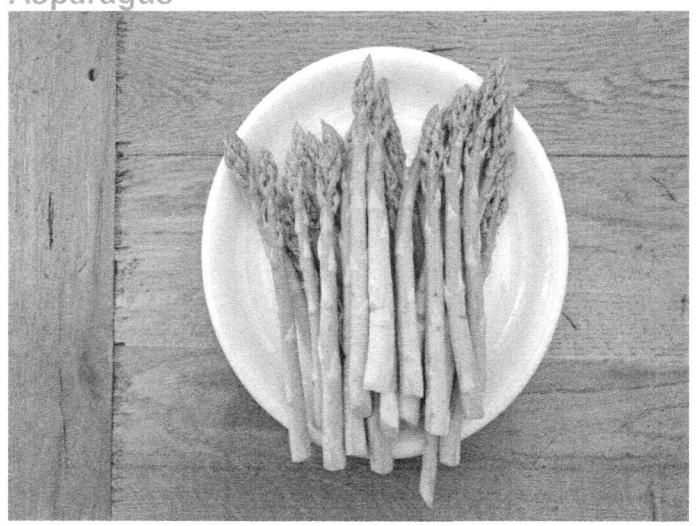

Asparagus is loaded with vitamins C, A, and K. It can help reduce strain and secure personality prosperity.

Mushrooms

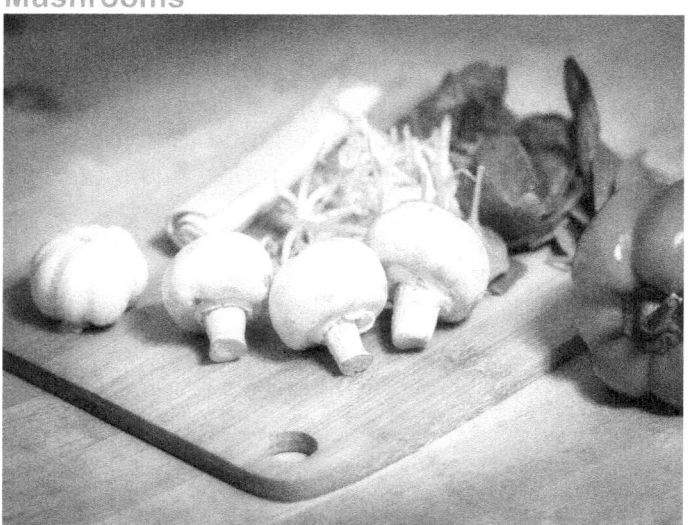

Mushrooms have exceptional alleviating properties. An examination shows that people who had metabolic turmoil have seen fundamental redesigns.

Squash
Many types of squash are high in sugar, and you should ensure that you pick the correct squash for your eating regimen. The best and most used is the mid-year squash. Summer squash is now and then utilized as a noodle substitution in dishes. It is high in fat and a marvelous side dish for your meal.

Spinach
Spinach contains vitamins and minerals. Additionally, it is heart friendly and reduces eye pains.

Avocado
It is high in fat, which makes it one of the best foods for a fat supplement. It is rich in Vitamin C and potassium.

Green Beans
Joined into the vegetable family, greens beans have fewer carbs than various conventional items. They are sometimes called snap peas. A measure of green beans just contains 6g net carbs, which makes them a splendid additional to any meal.

Cauliflower

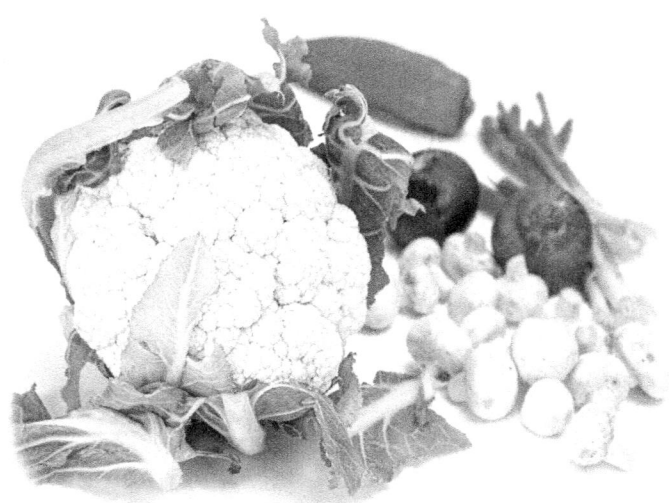

Known as the star of dishes, cauliflower is a versatile setting that can be added to different kinds of dinners. It can be used for pizzas, wraps, suppers and pureed potatoes. With only 2g net sugars for each glass, it is not surprising that cauliflower is a champion among the most consistently used fixings in some low-starch diets.

Kale and Lettuce

Used in servings of blended greens far and wide, kale and lettuce are low-sugar electives. They are a beautiful wellspring of Vitamins A and C and can help cut down the threats of heart infections.

Regardless of the fact that kale is more nutritious than lettuce, it has more carbs per serving. Consequently, be wary of how much kale you eat as sugars can incorporate speedily.

Do Not Eat

Grains

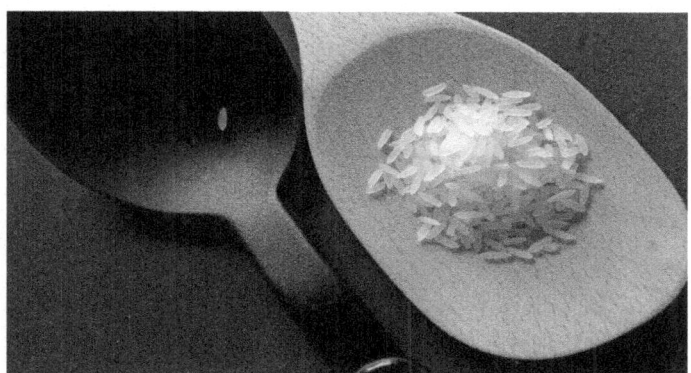

Swear off eating grains like rice, wheat and oats.

Sugars

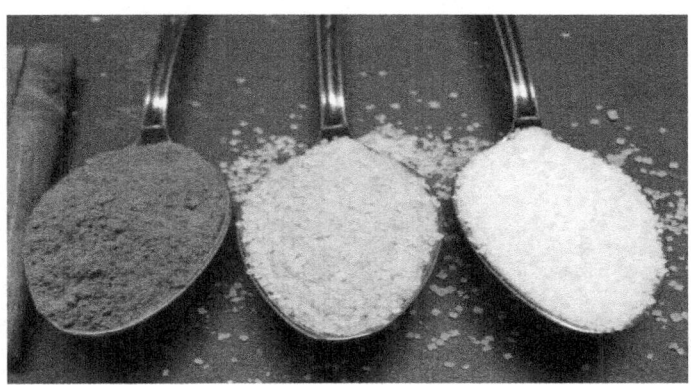

Your sugar intake should be kept to a base.

Stay away from eating sweets, nectar, maple syrup, even dark-hued sugar.

Tubers

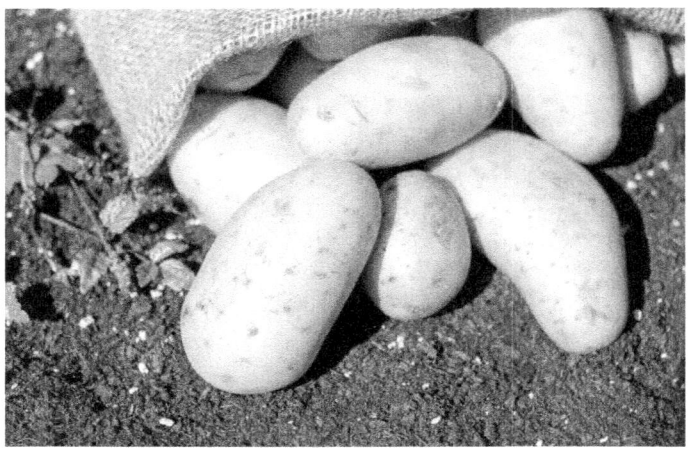

Do whatever it takes not to eat yams, potatoes, etc.

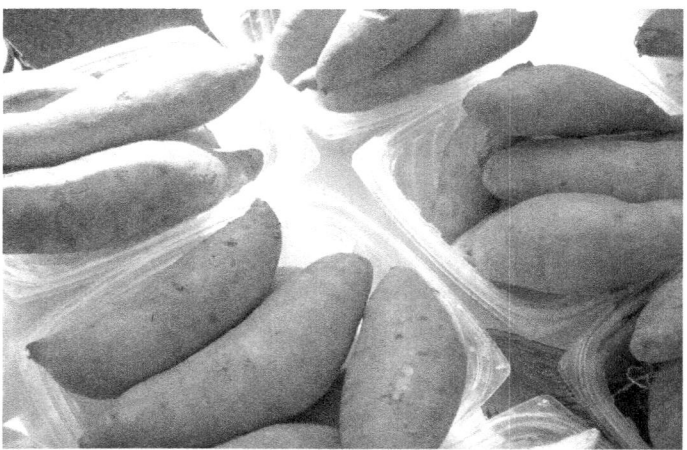

Natural items - Keep up a vital separation from or potentially control your use of essential things like bananas, apples, melons, etc.

Chapter 5: Dangers and Side Effects of the Ketogenic Diet and How to Avoid Them

Keto Flu

Ketone dieters who transition to a fat-burning mode may experience first side effects, such as nausea, headache, cramps, mood swings, etc. — also known as the Keto Flu. Here are some things you can do to help alleviate these symptoms:

Gradual reduction of carbs – You can prepare for a ketone diet by gradually reducing your intake of carbohydrates. A sudden drop in carb intake can shock your system, which can make you feel very uncomfortable.

A body that is not used to a low-carb diet will take the time to adjust. The sudden removal or dramatic decrease in carbohydrates will make the brain function with weaker energy. Once the body has adapted to the diet and to being fueled by ketones, said side effects disappear. A cup or two of bouillon daily is supposed to minimize the uncomfortable side effects of a ketone diet efficiently.

Bad Breath

Dieters who engage in a ketone diet or any low-carb diet can experience bad breath. This smell comes from acetone, which is a ketone body. The aroma is usually described as something fruity or like a nail polish remover. Now, although the term fruity seems right, it is not; otherwise, it would not be called as bad breath. It means that your body is turning into a fat burning machine and is creating ketones to fuel the body and the brain. This odor can also be a body odor that usually reveals itself when you exercise or sweat a lot.

It is worth noting that some people do not experience these symptoms. Others who suffer these temporary symptoms notice that they disappear once the body has adapted to the diet. Here are some more things to consider:

1. Drink More Water

It is usual to experience a dry mouth when you first engage in any low-carb diet. It is also a regular part of getting into ketosis. It results in having less saliva to clean away the bacteria in your mouth, which can lead to severe breath. Therefore, make sure to drink enough fluid and keep yourself hydrated. Salt is also an excellent cleansing ingredient.

2. Oral Hygiene

Maintaining good oral health is essential, especially when doing a keto diet. Although brushing your teeth will not get rid of the foul smell, it can help minimize it by preventing it from mixing with other unpleasant odors.

3. Breath Freshener

A breath freshener can be applied instantly and can somehow mask the smell of keto lingering in your breath.

4. Give it more time

In most cases, this kind of evil breath is only temporary, so just give it more time

If it does not go away after a few weeks or a month, an excellent way to deal with it is by reducing your level of ketosis. You can do this by eating more carbs. Usually, people can get out of ketosis by adding 50-70g of carbs — so only add a little bit. You can also combine this with intermittent fasting.

Leg cramps

Experiencing leg cramps is common when starting a keto diet. Although leg cramps do not usually pose much of a problem, they can be an issue when they become painful. Leg cramps are caused by the loss of magnesium because of increased urination. Here are three effective ways to prevent or cure leg cramps.

Salt and Water

The magical mixture of seawater can again be used to treat and prevent leg cramps. Be sure to drink enough fluid and keep yourself hydrated. This can also help you lower the loss of magnesium.

Magnesium Supplement

Since leg cramps are caused by the loss of magnesium, it is only logical to treat it by taking magnesium tablets.

Eat more carbs

As a last resort, you can increase your intake of carbohydrates. Take note, however, that this will weaken the effects of your ketone diet.

High Cholesterol Level

There is something dangerous about the Keto Diet taking a position that encourages consumption of foods that are high in fat. Although a low-carb, high-fat diet such as the Keto Diet is known for improving a dieter's cholesterol profile, a few people may experience some troubling results. It happens when the amount of good cholesterol exceeds the average level. Here are some things you can do to avoid this:

Lower your fat intake

Since consuming too much high fat is the cause of this problem, try to lower your fat intake, especially when you are not feeling hungry. Also, choose drinks that have lower fat content.

Intermittent Fasting

Intermittent fasting is like fasting, but it is only for a short period. It is an excellent way to lower your cholesterol level. For example, skip your breakfast, or merely eat just a little. You do not have to do this every day.

Alcoholic Beverages and Intoxication

It is not hard to notice that you can quickly become intoxicated when you follow a ketone diet or any low-carb diet. It is most likely due to the liver being busy creating ketones, so it could not function entirely to digest the liquor. But, the reason behind this remains unclear. In any case, once you engage in a Ketogenic Diet, you should be ready to deal with less alcohol tolerance. It is an excellent way to be healthy.

A problem with alcoholic drinks can be the carbs they contain, which is not okay for a Keto Diet. Therefore, you should choose your poison wisely.

If you want a touch of drink, the Bloody Mary is an excellent choice with only 7g of carbs, while a glass of margarita has 8g of carbs and Cosmopolitan has 13g of carbs. Not all drinks are prepared the same way, so be sure to check the carbs of your glass (usually written on the bottle or can), or just ask the bartender. Champagne is also an excellent choice with only 1g of carb per serving.

Keto Rash
Wear clothes that are comfortable and appropriate for the climate. Wearing less or thick clothing is recommended for sweating.

Use air conditioning or an electric fan, so you will not sweat. Keto Rash happens when ketones are released as you sweat followed by the drying up of the sweat on your skin.

You can choose either to partake in training programs that will make you perspire less or skip exercising all together. Especially if you just want to lose weight, walking and lightweight training are good options

Give it more time

If all else fails, the best way is to consult your doctor or just exit the state of ketosis. You can safely exit ketosis by gradually adding more carbs to your diet. If you wish to lose weight, adding around 50g-100g of carbs is usually enough to exit ketosis, but still good enough to make you forget weight. However, do not expect losing weight as fast as when you are in a state of ketosis.

Although the ketone diet can be used in the long-term, you are also free to do it for a short-term period. Either way, there can come a time when you only want to just wholly enjoy and not follow any strict diet program. Getting out of ketosis is easy: Just gradually add carbs to your diet.

There are people who had trouble with Keto Rash the first time they entered ketosis but found it to be less of a problem the second time they came into ketosis. Other times, the Keto Rash does not even appear the second time you come into ketosis. Therefore, if you are serious about going on a Keto Diet, it is best to give it another attempt so that you can enjoy the compelling benefits of the right Ketogenic Diet for you.

Drawbacks

As mentioned earlier, the Ketogenic Diet is not rid of its own set of disadvantages. Some of the challenges of the Ketogenic Diets include:

1. Low-Energy Levels: People who work in jobs that require high levels of energy or athletes may face challenges on starting the Ketogenic Diet because of the reduced energy levels.
2. Restrictive Eating: You can't eat whatever you please on this diet, as there are rules
3. Metabolic Problems: Critics also believe that going on a low-carb diet for an extended period may upset healthy metabolic function.

Some people also tend to overdo the low-carb thing.

Effects of the Ketogenic Diet

How the Body Utilizes Various Fuels

In the human body, there are three primary storage 'depots' of fuel that can be tapped into for supply of energy when there is a caloric deficiency.

The body would tap into its protein storage and convert it to glucose in the liver.

The body can draw into its carbohydrate (glycogen) store.

The body can also make use of its fat storage, which is stored in the body as body fat.

There is also a fourth type of fuel which the body can use, known as ketones. In an average diet, the ketones are insignificant to the body for energy production. However, on a low-carbohydrate diet such as the Ketogenic Diet, ketones are used a lot as a source of energy, especially by the brain.

Body tissues always make use of the most available source of fuel in the bloodstream. For instance, if there is a high concentration of glucose in the body, the body chooses glucose as its most preferred source of fuel except for organs like the heart that make use of a mixture of glucose, ketones and free fatty acids for fuel.

If, however, there is a reduction of the concentration of glucose in the body, the body will have to choose the next available source of fuel as its source of energy. On a Ketogenic Diet, the body switches from using glucose as its primary source of fuel to making use of stored fats due to the increased availability of fats in the body.

One of the goals of a Ketogenic Diet, therefore, is to increase the concentration of proteins and fats in the body as opposed to carbohydrates so that the body can switch to burning fat for energy which also will burn the excess fat stored in the body.

There are some other factors apart from fuel concentration that contribute to determining which fuels will be used by the body. They include levels of insulin and glucagon hormones in the body and levels of regulatory enzymes for breakdown of glucose and fats.

The process by which these ketones are formed is what is known as ketogenesis, and to understand the Ketogenic Diet, it is vital for you to grasp the concept of ketogenesis entirely. Ketogenesis in the body depends on two major factors: the liver and the fat cells.

As insulin levels in the blood reduce, mobilization of free fatty acids improves. It travels through the bloodstream aided by a protein known as Albumin, and, when it is in the blood, it can be used for energy production. Free fatty acids that are not used as fuel would be oxidized in the liver.

This oxidization leads to the production of ketone bodies, which are then released back into the bloodstream.

Along with the fat cells, the liver is another critical factor that determines ketogenesis in the body. The liver always produces ketones, whether on a Ketogenic Diet or not, but in small and hardly significant quantities.

The Ketogenic Diet, however, increases amounts of ketones present in the body. So, when people tell you ketones are harmful byproducts, remind them that ketones are always present in the body.

The liver is very essential for ketogenesis because, even if there are high levels of free fatty acids in the body, there would be no production of ketones if the liver is not in a ketogenic 'mood.'

The liver glycogen's primary function is to help maintain healthy glucose levels. When you are on a low-carb diet, and the blood glucose levels are reduced, the liver glycogen prompts the liver to break down its glycogen stores and release glucose into the bloodstream.

Your body makes use of this glucose for some time (between 12 and 16 hours depending on levels of physical activities), after which its glycogen stores become depleted. Upon depletion, ketogenesis increases rapidly according to the availability of free fatty acids.

Metabolic Effects of the Ketogenic Diet

One thing that critics are always quick to shout when the Ketogenic Diet is mentioned is that "the Ketogenic Diet will mess up your metabolism."

So, will the Ketogenic Diet mess up your metabolism?

Your metabolic system is primarily meant to make fuels available in your body whenever they are needed. As you continue to consume foods, your metabolic system continues to work to ensure that the energy from the foods are appropriately allocated, and then the excesses are stored.

The average human today eats too much, and, as a result, the metabolic system has to cope with more work than it is designed to handle.

During the starvation diet, the metabolic system focuses on the provision of glucose for tissues that necessarily require glucose to function such as the brain, kidney, red blood cells, etc. This glucose is usually obtained from the body's protein stores; mainly the muscles and sometimes from fat.

Your metabolic system doesn't know how long this starvation is going to continue; maybe for a few hours or a few weeks?

It first tries to cope with the situation by plundering the glucose supply in the blood and then takes some proteins from the muscles. But because it must also ensure that muscle mass is not excessively depleted, it turns to the ketones for a solution.

Ketones can stand in for glucose and proteins, so the muscles are spared from depletion, and your body is happy with using its new-found source of fuel – ketones – for energy.

It is what happens on a starvation diet, but with a low-carb diet; you would be eating some proteins and fats, so your muscles need not be depleted; the proteins you consume are converted to glucose.

So, will this diet ruin your metabolism?

Thermic Effect of Food:

This energy breaks down the macronutrients from consumed foods and processes them. Protein makes use of the highest amount of energy to be given out. It is why low-carb diets improve metabolism, but the same thing would happen with any food that increases consumption of protein and not just the Ketogenic Diet.

Thermic Effect of Activity:

This refers to any form of activity that is not a necessary body function such as exercises. People who are physically inactive and live sedentary lifestyles may only burn 10-30 percent more calories over their BMR, but physically active individuals who exercise regularly would consume more.

So, you see, it's not only what you eat that affects your metabolism. As long as you maintain a moderate level of physical activity and avoid complete starvation, you would be able to support a healthy metabolism.

What Not to Expect From the Ketogenic Diet

The diet is not a miracle weight loss solution or a yo-yo diet. It is a lifestyle change that takes a lot of discipline and hard work on your part to make it work. However, once you get used to the rudiments of the diet, you would begin to enjoy it and lose the weight very quickly.

You also shouldn't expect this diet to work without exercise. For better weight loss results, you should do the Ketogenic Diet along with regular exercise.

Chapter 6: How to Attain Ketosis

At the point when your liver separates fat, glycerol and unsaturated fat particles are created. The unsaturated fats are then divided further in a procedure alluded to as ketogenesis, and a ketone body alluded to as acetoacetate is then delivered. Acetoacetate is changed over into two sorts of ketone bodies.

Beta-hydroxybutyrate-Acetoacetate is ordinarily changed over into this ketone body when you have been on the Ketogenic Diet less for quite a while. Your mind leans towards this ketone.

Acetone: This might be processed into glucose; even though it is discharged as waste. It often causes a particular rank breath.

After some time, the body ousts fewer ketone bodies, and you may begin believing that ketosis is presumably backing off; this is not the situation. The cerebrum is consuming the beta-hydroxybutyrate, and your body is doing its best to give the mind however much vitality as could reasonably be expected. It is the reason that, if you are on the Ketogenic Diet for some time, you won't encounter profound levels of ketosis.

How to Know that You're in Ketosis

Measuring Ketones

To accomplish ketosis, you need serum ketones in the vicinity of 0.5 and 3.0mM. The following are easy to use home packs that can help you determine your ketone levels.

Breathalyzer

As specified before, when on a Ketogenic Diet, your breath has a particular scent. A breathalyzer is a shabby approach to quantify the centralization of CH3)2CO. Remember however that breath ketones can change with blood ketones.

Pee Ketone Strips

Ketostix and other pee recognition strips may not be as lucky because they just demonstrate the overabundance of ketone bodies being discharged from the body through urine. Be that as it may, they are easy to use.

Perception

You can tune into your body and decide whether you are in ketosis. For example, when in ketosis, your breath, pee and sweat notice CH3)2CO, which is a "fruity" odor. If you distinguish this, at that point, you are likely in ketosis.

With that comprehension of what happens to your body amid ketosis, the inquiry you might need to ask is; how at that point do you begin the eating routine?

Chapter 7: Useful Tips to Get the Most Out of the Ketogenic Diet

To get the best results in the shortest amount of time possible, get tips from the pros on the Ketogenic Diet, and how to integrate it into your life in a complete way.

Reading Nutrition Labels

Let's break nutrition labels down into parts. For this section, I'll be talking about U.S. food labels. First, the name tells you the serving size. If the serving size is "one packet," then go ahead and assess the rest of the nutrition label as is. But if the serving size is 2 per package, keep in mind that you need to either eat half of what you are holding or multiply everything by two.

The rest of the nutrition label should outline the carbohydrates, fats and proteins, along with other nutritional information. For the sugars, remember to subtract the dietary fiber from the total carbs to get your net carbs. Look for foods high in saturated or unsaturated fats but stay away from trans and hydrogenated fats. Protein, as usual, should be a medium amount of your intake.

Tips to Eat More Good Fat

If you try to get all the fat in your diet from fatty meats, you may find that your ratio of fat to protein quickly goes the wrong way. Keep in mind that a high-protein diet can lead to glucose in the bloodstream, knocking you out of ketosis. It's essential to supplement your meat intake with other forms of healthy fats.

So, what are some sneaky ways to increase your fat intake? Try piling avocado on top of your dishes. Make oil-thick salad dressings. Cook your vegetables in full-fat butter. Cook your plants in a tablespoon of coconut oil. Coconut oil, vegetable oils, butter, lard and healthy plant-based fats, like avocado, will all help improve your ratio of protein to fat in your diet, and they will also fill you up at mealtime.

Sleeping During Ketosis

One side effect of ketosis can often be insomnia, or the inability to sleep. It happens because of the lack of carbohydrates entering the body. Of course, carbs give us energy, but they also provide us dietary sources of tryptophan, a chemical that relaxes us and helps us sleep. Without this, it becomes harder to get a good night's rest.

You can offset this Keto insomnia by taking a tryptophan supplement. It may not fix the problem right away, but it should help over time. Other things that can help are increased mindfulness and meditation, as well as high levels of exercise.

Ketogenic Diet and Stress

There is a misinformed argument out there that the Ketogenic Diet causes stress within the body. This case is based on some misunderstandings of the core science of the body. Some people believe that when your body undergoes stress, you produce cortisol, and this cortisol can knock you out of ketosis.

The mistake comes next. Some think that GNG requires cortisol, or that cortisol promotes gluconeogenesis, but, in short, that's just not true. High levels of cortisol can trigger GNG, but GNG does not trigger the release of cortisol. In a nutshell, going into GNG does not add stress to your body.

Tips for Eating Out while on the Ketogenic Diet

Eating out in restaurants can be very challenging if you have a high-carb intolerance or coeliac disease. A great technique to dine at restaurants and still reduce unwanted pounds is to make better selections. Making more healthy choices is easier when dieters plan through researching guidebooks, which provide information on the nutrition content of meal options available at dining establishments. A fantastic place for finding this information is surfing the web. Some sites furnish these guides at no cost.

Here are five tips for eating out while on the Ketogenic Diet:

1. Conduct extensive research. You'll find a lot of restaurant reviews from low-carb bloggers on the internet, and you can also find information about which restaurants are gluten free on websites such as "The List" or "Urban Spoon".

2) Take a look at some restaurant menus on the internet - some restaurants use a lot of high-carb ingredients, whereas other restaurants don't use as much. Consider avoiding restaurants that use lots of flour, pastry, bread and other gluten containing ingredients.

3) Remember to tell your waiter or waitress that you require low-carb food, even if the menu in the restaurant has a low-carb section in it.

4) Double check everything - you can't be too careful when eating out in restaurants on the Ketogenic Diet. If you are served a meal that is obviously high in carbs, such as salad croutons, or bread on the plate, then be sure to send it back and ask for a fresh one.

5) Eating Keto at restaurants is a lot easier than you expect, once you get over the funny looks you might get from the waiter and your non-Keto friends.

Chapter 8: Breakfast Recipes

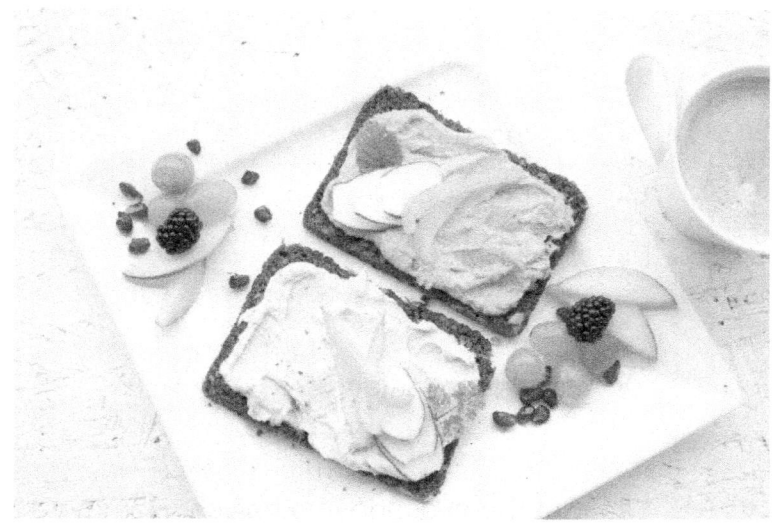

1. Avocado Stuffed with Tuna

Preparing time: 20 minutes

Serves: 6

Ingredients:

- 1 avocado
- 1 can of tuna
- 1 tomato
- ½ onion
- Parsley to taste

Directions:

1. Cut the avocado into halves. Remove the middle parts, so you can have a room for stuffing. (Keep the "meat" parts)
2. Cut the tomato and onion into tiny circles.
3. Mix meat parts with tuna, tomato, and onion.
4. Stuff the avocado halves with the mixture, decorate with parsley to taste and serve!

Nutritional Information Per Serving
(Calories: 132 | Fats: 3g | Net Carbs: 6g | Protein: 1.2g | Fiber: 7g)

2. Tuna in Cucumber

Preparing time: 15 minutes

Serves: 6

Ingredients:

- 1 cucumber
- ½ celery leaf
- ½ red bell pepper
- 1 can of tuna
- Pepper and salt to taste

Directions:

1. Peel the cucumber and cut it into thicker circles. Make a hole in each piece.
2. Cut the celery and pepper into tiny cubes. Mix them with tuna.
3. Put 1 tbsp. of tuna mixture into cucumbers.
4. Add spices to taste and serve.
5. Enjoy!

Nutritional Information Per Serving
(Calories: 109 | Total Fats: 1.6g | Net Carbs: 4g | Protein: 1g |Fiber: 5.4g)

3. Small Keto Pies

Preparing time: 25 Minutes

Serves: 6

Ingredients:

- 3 eggs
- 5 bacon slices
- ½ red bell pepper
- 1 leek
- ½ cup of broccoli
- 2 oz. of ground cheese
- ½ cup of yogurt
- ¼ pack of baking powder
- 2 tbsp. of olive oil
- Salt, pepper, powdered garlic, parsley to taste

Directions:

1. Whisk and blend the eggs with baking powder.
2. Cook the broccoli in water.

3. Cut bacon, leek and pepper into smaller pieces to taste.

4. Mix cheese with yogurt well. Then, add bacon, leek, pepper, and spices to taste.

5. Join the 2 mixtures together and then pour into cupcake or muffin molds.

6. Bake for 30 minutes at 200°F.

Nutritional Information Per Serving
(Calories: 121 | Total Fats: 2.1g | Net Carbs: 2g | Protein: 1.3g | Fiber: 6g)

4. Keto Wraps

Preparing time: 30 minutes

Serves: 6

Ingredients:

- 10 oz. of turkey meat
- 3 oz. of bacon
- 1 tomato
- 3 oz. of mozzarella
- Cabbage leaves for wrapping

For coating:

- 1 cup of mayonnaise
- 6 basil leaves
- 1 tsp. of lemon juice
- 1 tsp. of powdered garlic
- 1 tsp. of salt
- 1 tsp. of pepper

Directions:

1. Mix all ingredients listed for coating in one bowl. You should get a dense mixture.
2. Prepare bacon in a frying pan.

3. Coat cabbage leaves with coating mixture. Pile ingredients over (turkey, tomatoes, bacon and cheese).

4. Wrap the cabbage like tortillas and serve.

Nutritional Information Per Serving
(Calories: 121 | Total Fats: 6.9g | Net Carbs: 4g | Protein: 2.4g |Fiber: 5.6g)

5. Chicken Omelet

Preparing time: 15 minutes

Serves: 1

Ingredients:

- 1 oz. of rotisserie chicken, shredded
- 1 tsp. of mustard
- 1 tbsp. of mayonnaise
- 1 tomato, cored and chopped
- 2 bacon slices, cooked and crumbled
- 2 eggs
- 1 small avocado, pitted, peeled and chopped
- Salt and ground black pepper, to taste

Directions:

1. Heat up a pan over medium heat, grease lightly with cooking oil.
2. Mix the eggs with some salt and pepper in a bowl and whisk.

3. Add the eggs in the pan and cook the omelet for 5 minutes.

4. Add the chicken, avocado, tomato, bacon, mayonnaise and mustard on one half of the omelet.

5. Fold the omelet, cover pan, cook for 5 minutes and serve.

Nutritional Information Per Serving
(Calories: 400 | Total Fats: 32g | Net Carbs: 4g | Protein: 25g |Fiber: 6)

6. Eggs in Pepper

Preparing time: 25 Minutes

Serves: 3

Ingredients:

- 6 eggs
- 1 bell pepper, sliced into ¼ in. rings
- Salt and ground black pepper, to taste
- 2 tbsp. of chopped chives and parsley
- 2 tbsp. of olive oil

Directions:

1. Heat a frying pan to medium heat and grease it lightly.
2. Place bell pepper rings in the pan for 2 minutes.
3. Flip the rings and crack an egg in the middle of the rings.
4. Add salt and pepper.
5. Cook 2-4 minutes.

6. Repeat with other pepper rings and eggs.

7. Garnish with parsley and chives.

Nutritional Information Per Serving
(Calories: 157| Total Fats: 12g | Net Carbs: 6g | Protein: 12g |Fiber: 6.3g)

7. Naan Bread and Butter

Preparing time: 20 minutes

Serves: 6

Ingredients:

- 7 tablespoons coconut oil
- ¾ cup coconut flour
- 2 tablespoons psyllium powder
- ½ teaspoon baking powder
- Salt, to taste
- 2 cups hot water
- Some coconut oil, for frying
- 2 garlic cloves, peeled and minced
- 3. 5 ounces butter

Directions:

1. In a bowl, mix the coconut flour with baking powder, salt, and psyllium powder, and stir.
2. Add the coconut oil and the hot water and knead the dough. Set aside for 5 minutes, divide into 6 balls, and flatten them on a working surface.
3. Heat up a pan with some coconut oil over medium-high heat, add the naan

bread to the pan, fry them until golden brown, and transfer them to a plate.

4. Heat up a pan with the butter over medium-high heat, add the garlic, salt, and pepper, stir, and cook for 2 minutes.

5. Brush the naan bread with this mixture and pour the rest into a bowl and serve.

Nutritional Information Per Serving
(Calories: 140 | Total Fats: 9g | Net Carbs: 3g | Protein: 4g | Fiber: 1g)

8. Breakfast Tuna Salad

Preparing time: 10 minutes

Serves: 4

Ingredients:

- 2 tbsp. of sour cream
- 12 oz. of canned tuna in olive oil
- 4 leeks, diced
- A pinch of red chili flakes
- 1 tbsp. of capers
- 8 tbsp. of mayonnaise
- Salt and ground black pepper, to taste

Directions:

1. Mix all ingredients listed in one salad bowl.
2. Stir well and serve.

Nutritional Information Per Serving
(Calories: 160g| Total Fats: 3g | Net Carbs: 2g | Protein: 6g |Fiber:1g)

9. Deviled Eggs

Preparing time: 25 minutes

Serves: 6

Ingredients

- 3 eggs
- ½ cup of cream cheese
- Salt, to taste
- 1 tsp. of red pepper
- 10 olives

Directions:

1. Cook eggs in water. Peel them and cut into halves and remove the yolks.
2. Combine cooked yolks with cheese and olives (thinly cut). Blend them together nicely.
3. Stuff eggs with resulting mixture.
4. Serve with a salad to taste and enjoy!

Nutritional information Per Serving (Calories 89g | Total Fats 2.6g | Net Carbs: 6g | Protein 3g | Fiber: 2.6g)

10. Low-Carb Muffins with Whey

Preparing time: 45 minutes

Serves: 6

Ingredients:

- 1 egg
- 4 tsp. of whey (Chocolate)
- 4 tbsp. of low-fat milk
- 1 tsp. of cacao
- ½ tsp. of vanilla sugar
- ½ pack of baking powder

Directions:

1. In one bowl, whisk 1 egg with milk and vanilla sugar. Combine them well.
2. Gradually, add whey, cacao, and baking powder to the mixture. Mix constantly.
3. Pour resulting mixture into muffin molds.
4. Bake at 220°F for 30 minutes. Enjoy!

Nutritional Information Per Serving **(Calories: 112 | Total Fats: 5g | Net Carbs: 6g | Protein: 1.2g |Fiber: 3.3g)**

11. Spinach Rolls

Preparing time: 30 minutes

Serves: 6

Ingredients:

- 7 oz. of white meat, cut into small cubes
- 1 cup of spinach
- 4 eggs
- 7 oz. of cream cheese
- 1 tbsp. of sesame seeds
- ½ tsp. of sodium bicarbonate
- 4 tbsp. of flour

Directions:

1. Cook spinach and meat in water. (Separately)
2. Whisk 3 eggs with 4 tbsp. of flour, sodium, salt, 2 tbsp. of cheese and ½ cup of cooked spinach.

3. Mix them well and bake at 250°F for 10 minutes.

4. Meanwhile, dissolve a pinch of salt in water. Add ½ cup of cooked spinach, meat and 1 egg. Cook the mixture in a cooking pot until meat is done.

5. Cut baked dough into smaller sizes, fill them with cooked mixture and roll. Enjoy!

Nutritional Information Per Serving
(Calories: 123 | Total Fats: 4g | Net Carbs: 8g | Protein: 3g |Fiber: 2.4g)

12. Breakfast Smoothie

Preparing time: 5 minutes

Serves: 6

Ingredients:

- 1 banana
- ½ cup of frozen cherries
- 1 tbsp. of flax seeds
- 2 cups of milk

Directions:

1. Peel and cut the banana into smaller pieces.
2. Unfreeze the cherries naturally or in a cooking pot.
3. Put all ingredients in a blender and mix nicely for about 30 seconds. Enjoy!

Nutritional information Per Serving (Calories 111 | Total Fats 2.3g | Net Carbs: 4g | Protein 2.2g |Fiber: 3g)

13. Low-Carb Breakfast Balls

Preparing time: 25 minutes

Serves: 6

Ingredients:

- 7 oz. of chicken meat
- 3 oz. of cheese
- 1 tbsp. of sour cream
- 2 tbsp. of mayonnaise
- ½ cup of olives, ground
- Cheese for rolling

Directions:

1. Cook chicken meat in water. When it is done, cut it into very tiny pieces or grind it.
2. Combine meat with cheese, sour cream and mayonnaise.
3. Make small balls out of the mixture and then roll them into the cheese.
4. Serve and enjoy!

Nutritional Information Per Serving **(Calories: 123 | Total Fats: 2.5g | Net Carbs: 3g | Protein: 3.2g | Fiber: 2.3g)**

14. Keto Muffins with Chicken

Preparing time: 50 minutes

Serves: 6

Ingredients:

- 4 oz. of chicken fillets
- 2 eggs
- 3 tsp. of cheese
- 6 tsp. of oat flakes
- Spices, to taste

Directions:

1. Cut fillets into tiny pieces.
2. Separate egg yolks from egg whites.
3. Combine egg yolk with cheese, meat, flakes and spices.
4. Blend whites into dense cream.
5. Gradually, join 2 mixtures together.
6. Pour resulting mixture into muffin molds and bake for 20 minutes at 250°F.

Nutritional Information Per Serving
(Calories: 142 | Total Fats: 1.5g | Net Carbs: 3g | Protein: 2.1g |Fiber: 2g)

15. Borecole with Curry

Preparing time: 30 minutes

Serves: 6

Ingredients:

- 2 eggs
- 10 oz. of borecole
- Salt, pepper to taste
- 1 tbsp. of powdered curry

Directions:

1. Wash borecole and cut thinly. Cook in water for 10 minutes, so it becomes soft.
2. Whisk eggs with spices. Mix well.
3. Soak borecole into the egg mixture and put it on an oiled baking tray.
4. Bake for 15 minutes at 300°F.

   Nutritional Information Per Serving
   (Calories: 131 | Total Fats: 4g | Net Carbs: 5g | Protein: 3g |Fiber: 2g)

16. Eggs on Sour Cream

Preparing time: 35 minutes

Serves: 6

Ingredients:

- 6 eggs
- 1 cup of sour cream
- 1 tbsp. of parsley
- 1 tbsp. of butter
- Salt, to taste

Directions:

1. Spread sour cream over casserole dish equally.
2. Make 6 holes in the sour cream mixture and pour the egg into each one.
3. Add salt and parsley. Bake for 15 minutes at 250°F.

Nutritional Information Per Serving **(Calories: 98 | Total Fats: 2g | Net Carbs: 3g | Protein: 4g |Fiber: 5g)**

17. Low-Carb Bacon Muffins

Preparing time: 40 minutes

Serves: 6

Ingredients:

- 2 eggs
- 4 oz. of sour cream
- 2 oz. of butter
- 4 oz. of low-carb flour
- 4 oz. of cheese
- 4 oz. of bacon
- Salt, to taste

Directions:

1. Whisk the eggs. Combine them with melted butter, sour cream and flour. Mix well.
2. Cut bacon thinly. Grind the cheese and then combine these two.
3. Join 2 mixtures together and fill muffin molds with resulting combination.
4. Bake for 25 minutes at 220°F. Enjoy!

Nutritional Information Per Serving (Calories: 85 | Total Fats: 6g | Net Carbs: 7g | Protein: 2g |Fiber: 6g)

18. Zucchini in Yogurt

Preparing time: 15 minutes

Serves: 6

Ingredients:

- 1 zucchini
- 1 cup of yogurt
- Salt, pepper and oregano, to taste

Directions:

1. Cut zucchinis into circles. Pour salt over them and let them sit for 5 minutes.
2. Strain the water, and sauté zucchini circles in a frying pan. (Without oil)
3. Pour yogurt over zucchini and serve!

Nutritional Information Per Serving
(Calories: 109 | Total Fats: 3.5g | Net Carbs: 6g | Protein: 2.4g | Fiber: 4g)

19. Gluten-Free, Keto Coconut Bread

Preparing time: 10 minutes

Serves: 6

Ingredients:

- 2 eggs
- 1 tsp. of baking powder
- 2 tbsp. of coconut flour
- 2 tsp. of butter
- 1 tsp. of salt

Directions:

1. Whisk eggs and salt them.
2. Mix them with flour and baking powder.
3. Pour mixture into 2 ceramic cups.
4. Cook them in a microwave for 2 minutes at max heat.
5. Enjoy your ideal fast ketogenic bread!

Nutritional Information Per Serving **(Calories: 106 | Total Fats: 4g | Net Carbs: 5g | Protein: 5g | Fiber: 6g)**

20. Baked Brussels Sprout with Garlic

Preparing time: 35 minutes

Serves: 6

Ingredients:

- 14 oz. of Brussels sprout
- 1 tbsp. of powdered garlic
- ½ tsp. of chili pepper
- 4 tbsp. of olive oil
- Pinch of salt

Directions:

1. Cook brussels sprout in boiling water for 2 minutes.
2. Strain the water, add powdered garlic and pepper.
3. Sprinkle everything with olive oil and add salt.
4. Pour mixture into a casserole dish to bake for 25 minutes at 220°F.

Nutritional information Per Serving **(Calories: 131 | Total Fats: 5g | Net Carbs: 8g | Protein: 3g |Fiber: 5g)**

21. Ketogenic Protein Muffins

Preparing time: 25 minutes

Serves:6

Ingredients:

- 2 eggs
- 1 tbsp. of coconut flour
- 1 tbsp. of vanilla whey
- ½ cup of yogurt
- Stevia, to taste

Directions:

1. Whisk eggs and combine with yogurt, flour, whey, and stevia.
2. Fill muffin molds with resulting mixture.
3. Bake for 20 minutes at 250°F.
4. Serve and enjoy!

Nutritional Information Per Serving **(Calories: 114 | Total Fats: 6g | Net Carbs: 5g | Protein: 1.6g |Fiber: 4.7g)**

22. Fried Peppers with Cauliflowers

Preparing time: 55 minutes

Serves: 6

Ingredients:

- 1 onion
- 1 red bell pepper
- 1 yellow bell pepper
- 1 green bell pepper
- 2 tbsp. of olive oil
- 1 cup of cauliflowers
- Salt, pepper, powdered garlic to taste 3 eggs
- Parsley leaves

Directions:

1. Clean and cut all vegetables into tiny pieces. (Peppers and onion into cubes)
2. Blend cauliflowers.
3. Sauté onion and peppers in oil. When they become soft, add cauliflowers.

4. Add spices and fry for 4 minutes.

5. After that, add eggs and parsley. Cook for another 5 minutes and then serve.

Nutritional Information Per Serving
(Calories: 129 | Total Fats: 5.1g | Net Carbs: 4g | Protein: 1.7g |Fiber: 3.1g)

23. Eggs Sauce

Preparing time: 15 minutes

Serves: 6

Ingredients:

- 4 hard boiled eggs
- 2 tbsp. of oat flakes
- 4 tbsp. of sesame seeds
- 1 tbsp. of olive oil
- 5 slices of bacon
- Powdered garlic, chili, basil, salt to taste

Directions:

1. Mix all ingredients in a blender.
2. Mix them thinly.
3. Serve with ketogenic bread!

Nutritional Information Per Serving
(Calories: 132 | Total Fats: 6g | Net Carbs: 5g | Protein: 0.4g |Fiber: 1.6g)

24. Keto Breakfast

Preparing time: 15 minutes

Serves: 6

Ingredients:

- 1 tbsp. of butter
- ½ avocado
- 2 large portobello mushrooms
- 5 thin bacon slices
- 1 egg
- Salt, to taste
- Freshly ground black pepper

Directions:

1. Heat half the butter in a pan over medium heat.

2. Add mushrooms, sprinkle salt and pepper and cook for around 8 minutes, or until cooked.

3. Fry the bacon and egg in a separate pan, since the mushroom will release moisture.

4. Once ready, serve and enjoy.

Nutritional Information Per Serving (Calories: 234 | Total Fats: 41.3 g | Net Carbs: 6.6 g | Protein: 19.5 g | Fiber: 11.6g)

25. Bacon Burger

Preparing time: 45 minutes

Serves: 1

Ingredients:

- 2 tbsp. of cheddar cheese
- ¼ tsp. of Worcestershire
- ¼ tsp. of onion powder
- ½ tsp. of salt
- ¾ tsp. of soy sauce
- ½ tsp. of black pepper
- ½ tsp. of minced garlic
- 1 ½ tsp. of chopped chives
- 2 slices bacon
- 200g of ground beef

Directions:

1. Cook the bacon in a skillet until crisp.

2. Once ready, remove from the skillet, put on a paper towel, drain the grease and put aside.

3. Combine bacon, beef and spices in a large bowl.

4. Form three patties, then put 2 tbsp. of the bacon fat on the skillet.

5. Once the fat is hot, put the patties in the skillet and cook on each side for 4 minutes, or depending on preference.

6. Remove the patties from the skillet and allow to rest for 3 minutes.

7. Assemble the burger starting with one patty, then bacon and some cheese, another patty, bacon and cheese and the final patty on top.

Nutritional Information Per Serving **(Calories: 145 | Total Fats: 51.8g | Net Carbs: 1.8g | Protein: 43.5g | Fiber: 11.6g)**

26. Pesto Scrambled Eggs

Preparing time: 25 minutes

Serves: 1

Ingredients:

- 3 organic eggs
- Freshly ground black pepper
- Salt, to taste
- 2 tbsp. of sour cream
- 1 tbsp. of pesto
- 1 tbsp. of butter

Directions:

1. Beat eggs in a bowl and season with pepper and salt.

2. Heat a pan over medium heat, add butter; once hot, pour the eggs into the pan.

3. Cook on low heat and stir constantly. Add the pesto and mix.

4. Remove from heat, add cream and mix with eggs. It will make the eggs have a creamy mixture.

Nutritional Information Per Serving (Calories: 231 | Total Fats: 41.5g | Net Carbs: 2.6g | Protein: 20.4g | Fiber: 11.6g)

27. Keto Waffles with Pumpkin Spice

Preparing time: 35 minutes

Serves: 6

Ingredients:

- 1 tsp. of baking powder
- 1 tsp. of vanilla extract
- 3 tbsp. of swerve sweetener
- 1 ½ tsp. pumpkin pie spice
- ⅓ cup of coconut milk
- ½ cup of almond flour
- 2 tbsp. of flaxseed meal
- ¼ cup of canned pumpkin
- 2 large eggs
- 7 drops of liquid stevia

Directions:

1. Mix all of your wet ingredients in a large bowl. Be sure to mix well, until no egg whites are visible.

2. Combine all dry ingredients in a sifter.

3. If you don't have a sifter, just mixing all of the dry ingredients in a bowl and slowly sprinkling them into the wet ingredients will work too.

4. Combine the wet and dry ingredients until they are thoroughly combined.

5. Heat your waffle iron and grease. Coconut spray gives your waffles a vague hint of coconut!

6. Pour your mixture into the iron and cook until the built-in alarm goes off, or the stream of steam begins to dissipate. Serve with your favorite syrup!

Nutritional Information Per Serving (Calories: 30 | Total Fat: 2.5g | Net Carbs: 0.5g | Protein: 1.5g | Fiber: 11.6g)

28. Keto Cheese Tacos

Preparing time: 35 minutes

Serves: 6

Ingredients:

- 3 strips of bacon
- 1 oz. of cheddar cheese, shredded
- ½ avocado
- 2 tbsp. of butter
- 1 cup of mozzarella cheese, shredded
- 6 large eggs
- Salt and pepper, to taste

Directions:

1. Start by thoroughly cooking the bacon. Either in an oven for 15 to 20 minutes at 375°F or on the stovetop.

2. Heat a clean pan over medium heat and add ⅓ cup of mozzarella.

3. Cook the cheese until it begins to bubble and turn brown on the side touching the pan. Pay close attention here!

4. Slip a spatula under the cheese and gently unstick it from the pan.

5. Now use a pair of tongs and drape the cheese over a wooden spoon, that should be

resting over a bowl or pot. Allow the cheese to cool and form a taco shell shape.

6. Repeat Steps 2 to 5 with the rest of your mozzarella.

7. Now add your butter and eggs to the pan and cook thoroughly, adding salt and pepper to suit your taste.

8. Divide the eggs equally between your cheese shells.

9. Slice the avocado and divide the slices evenly between the tacos.

10. Chop or crumble your bacon, and divide equally between the tacos.

11. Sprinkle your cheddar cheese over the tops.

Nutritional Information Per Serving **(Calories: 30 | Total Fat: 2.5g | Net Carbs: 0.5g | Protein: 1.5g | Fiber: 11.6g)**

28. Keto Mini Doughnuts

Preparing time: 25 minutes

Serving size: 22

Ingredients:

- 4 tbsp. almond flour
- 1 tbsp. coconut flour
- 1 tsp. vanilla extract
- 1 tsp. baking powder
- 4 tbsp. erythritol
- 3 oz. cream cheese
- 3 large eggs
- 10 drops liquid stevia

Directions:

1. Combine with an immersion blender or a food processor.

2. Make sure that all your ingredients are well blended and smooth.

3. Heat your doughnut maker and spray with your grease of choice. Coconut oil always gives your cooking a delicious finish!

4. Pour your mixture into the doughnut maker. Leave some room (say 10%) to give your doughnuts space to rise.

5. Let the mixture cook for 3 minutes, and then flip and cook for an additional 2 minutes.

6. Remove the baked doughnuts and repeat Steps 3 to 5 for the rest of your batter.

Voilà! You've just created 22 good keto-friendly donuts.

Nutritional Information Per Serving **(Calories: 30 | Total Fat: 2.5g | Net Carbs: 0.5g | Protein: 1.5g | Fiber: 11.6g)**

29. Chive and Bacon Omelet

Preparing time: 35 minutes

Serves: 6

Ingredients:

- 1 oz. of cheddar cheese
- 1 tsp. of bacon fat
- 2 slices of bacon (cooked)
- 2 stalks of cheddar
- 2 large eggs
- Salt and pepper, to taste

Directions:

1. Make sure your chives are chopped, cheese shredded, eggs are cracked and mixed and bacon cooked before you begin.

2. Heat your bacon fat in a pan on medium-low heat.

3. Add your eggs, chives and salt and pepper to the pan.

4. Cook until you can see the edges start to set, and then cook for another 30 seconds.

5. Immediately add your bacon to the center of the omelet, and turn off the heat.

6. Sprinkle your cheese on top of the bacon.

7. Fold two edges of the egg on top of the bacon/cheese pile. The melted cheese should hold the egg in place.

8. Repeat Step 7 with the rest of the egg. It will create a slightly burrito shaped omelet.

9. Flip the egg over and allow it to cook a little longer in the pan (it'll still be warm).

10. Feel free to sprinkle some extra chive, cheese or bacon on top.

Nutritional Information Per Serving **(Calories: 321 | Total Fat: 36g | Net Carbs: 2g | Protein: 25g | Fiber: 11.6g)**

30. Baked Avocados with Eggs and Bacon

Preparing time: 35 minutes

Serves: 6

Ingredients:

- 2 small eggs
- 2 slices of bacon
- 1 avocado
- Pepper, to taste

Directions:

1. Pan fry your bacon until it is just barely cooked.

2. Pre-heat your oven to 425°F.

3. Halve the avocado and remove the pit.

4. Crumple some aluminum foil into ring shapes that will hold your avocado halves up on the baking sheet.

5. Break your eggs into a bowl, and spoon one yolk into each avocado half. Then continue to fill the hole of each avocado with egg whites until they're both full.

6. Crumble your bacon and spread on top of the avocados.

7. Add pepper on top and bake in the preheated oven for 12 to 15 minutes.

8. After 10 minutes, check your eggs every minute or two to ensure you don't overcook them.

Serve them up!

Nutritional Information Per Serving (**Calories: 98 | Total Fat: 60g | Net Carbs: 6g | Protein: 23g | Fiber: 11.6g**)

Chapter 9: Lunch Recipes

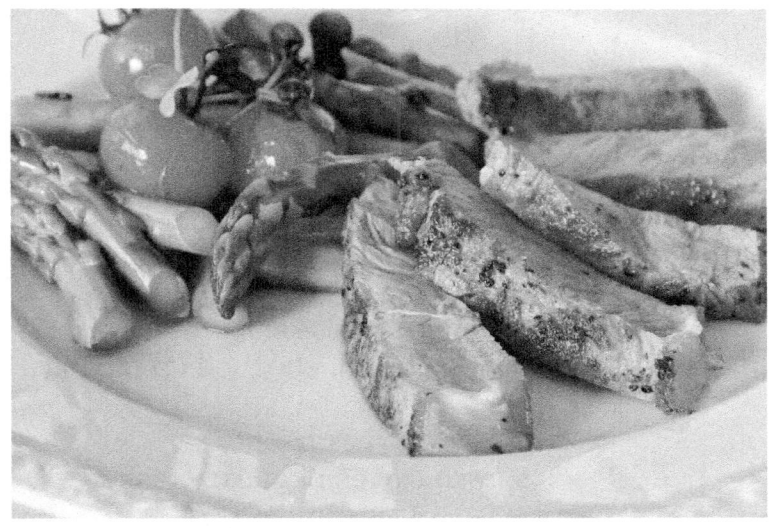

31. Beef Burritos

Preparing time: 35 minutes

Serves: 8

Ingredients:

Beef:
- 2 lbs. of sirloin steak
- 1 cup of chicken soup or broth (canned works well)
- 1 cup of BBQ sauce
- ½ of an onion, chopped up roughly
- 2 tsp. of salt
- ½ tsp. of black pepper
- 5 fresh cloves of garlic, crushed
- ½ tsp. of cinnamon
- 2 bay leaves

Taco:
- 8 low-carb wraps
- ½ cup of mayo
- 1 ½ cups of coleslaw (you can make your own, but ready bought works just as well)

Prepping Advice:
- Prepare the filling in advance
- Add to the tacos on the day.

Directions:

1. Pat dry the sirloin with paper towels, and score along the sides.
2. Combine the salt, pepper and cinnamon. Sprinkle it evenly onto the steak, making sure that there is an even covering.
3. Put the onion and garlic in the slow cooker. Place the beef on top and cover with the soup. Add the bay leaves and cook for eight hours.
4. When cooked, remove and strain the ingredients. Then shred the beef mix by pulling it with two forks.
5. Add the BBQ sauce and combine everything well.
6. Put some of the beef into the wrap, add coleslaw and dash of mayo. Wrap and eat.

Nutritional Information Per Serving
(Calories: 750 | Total Fat: 50g | Net Carbs: 14g | Protein: 60g | Fiber: 7.3g)

32. Open-Faced Prosciutto and Brie Sandwich with Avocado Bun

Preparing time: 35 minutes

Serves: 8

Ingredients:

- 1 avocado
- 4 small slices of brie
- 8 thin slices of prosciutto
- 6 mushrooms (any variety, but large flat ones work well)
- 2 cups of raw spinach
- 2 tsp. of butter
- Pinch of sesame seeds
- Pinch of salt
- Sprinkle of black pepper

Prepping Advice:

- Measure out the ingredients in advance.
- Cook up on the day you will be eating the sandwich.

Directions:
1. Cook the spinach for five minutes until it has wilted. Drain and squeeze out excess water.
2. Slice the mushroom and sauté in the butter until soft. Add some pepper and salt.

3. Cut the avocado in half. Cut a slice off the bottom of one half of the avocado, so it can stand. This will be your 'bottom slice of bread'.
4. Fill the two halves of your avocado with the ingredients. Serve as open-faced sandwich

Nutritional Information Per Serving
(Calories: 65 | Total Fat: 40g | Net Carbs: 12g | Protein: 16g | Fiber: 7.3g)

33. The Keto Cubano

Preparing time: 25 minutes

Serves: 8

Ingredients:

- Thinly sliced dill pickles or ready-made pickles of your choice
- ⅓ lb. of thinly sliced cooked ham
- ⅓ lb. of cooked pork tenderloin
- ¼ pound of sliced swiss cheese
- 1 tbsp. of melted butter or coconut oil to put on the paninis.
- 2 tbsp. of mayonnaise
- 2 tbsp. Dijon mustard
- Low-carb wraps or bib lettuce

Prepping Advice:

- Measure out the ingredients in advance.
- Cook on the day.

Directions:
1. Mix the mayo and mustard together and spread over the wrap (if using low-carb wrap)

2. Divide up the pickle, cheese and meats between the sandwiches. Roll up the wraps tightly.
3. Place in a sandwich maker, or in a panini press and cook for 5 to 7 minutes.
4. If using the lettuce instead of the wraps, simply omit Step 3.

Nutritional Information Per Serving
(Calories: 235 | Total Fat: 36g | Net Carbs: 7g | Protein: 28g | Fiber: 7.3g

34. Keto Monkey Bread

Preparing time: 45 minutes

Serves: 6

Ingredients:

- 2 baby eggplants, cubed
- ¾ cup of mozzarella cheese, shredded
- 2 tbsp. of melted butter
- 1 tbsp. of fresh basil, chopped roughly into small pieces
- 1 clove of garlic, crushed

Prepping Advice

- Cook in advance and reheat.

Directions:

1. Pre-heat the oven to 375°F.
2. Take a muffin pan and lightly grease.
3. Combine the garlic, melted butter and a half of the basil.
4. Place some of the eggplant (four or five pieces) into the bottom of each muffin tray.
5. Sprinkle even amounts of mozzarella and drizzle

butter mixture over each portion of eggplant.
6. Add the remaining cheese on top and bake for around 20 minutes. The cheese should be nicely browned.
7. Allow to cool for 5 minutes and eat warm; you can reheat later.

Nutritional Information Per Serving (Calories: 195 | Total Fat: 15g | Net Carbs: 6g | Protein: 8g | Fiber: 7.3g)

35. Beef Stew

Preparing time: 35 minutes

Serves: 8

Ingredients:

- 1 ½ lbs. of stewing beef cut into cubes (or, you can always go for a better cut, such as sirloin)
- 2 cans of chopped tomatoes
- 1 tbsp. of chili mix – a ready-made bought one is fine
- 1 cup of beef broth
- 2 tsp. of a hot chili sauce (optional)
- 1 tbsp. of Worcestershire sauce
- Salt, to taste

Prepping Advice:

- Cook the meal at prepping time, and reheat as required

Directions:
1. Turn the slow cooker on to low.
2. Put in all the ingredients in and give a mix.
3. Cook for 8 hours.
4. Add salt, to taste

Nutritional Information Per Serving
(Calories: 222 | Total Fat: 7g | Net Carbs: 9g | Protein: 27g | Fiber: 7.3g)

36. Beef Welly

Preparing time: 30 minutes

Serves: 8

Ingredients:

- 2 tenderloin steaks (hint: don't skimp on the beef. Go for best quality, it will pay dividends)
- 1 tbsp. of butter
- 4 tbsp. of liver pâté
- 1 cup of mozzarella cheese
- ½ cup of almond flour
- Salt and pepper, to taste

Prepping Advice:

- Measure out the ingredients.
- This can be reheated, but for such a special dish, it is best enjoyed fresh.

Directions:
1. Season the steaks to taste.
2. Melt the butter in a pan so that it is sizzling, but not burning. Put the steaks in the pan.
3. Sear all sides, then take the steaks off the heat and allow them to cool.
4. Heat the mozzarella in the microwave for about a minute.
5. Stir in the almond flour while the cheese is still hot. It will form a dough.

6. Place the dough, while still as warm as possible, between two pieces of grease proof paper and roll flat.
7. Place a tablespoon of pâté, about the size that the meat will cover, onto the dough. Spread it out so that it will encircle the meat.
8. Cut the dough so it will form a complete ball around the meat, when added, and the pâté.
9. Put a piece of meat inside the dough, cut it and wrap it around the meat and pâté.
10. Repeat for the other piece of meat.

Nutritional Information Per Serving
(Calories: 307 | Total Fat: 22g | Net Carbs: 2.5g | Protein: 26g | Fiber: 7.3g)

37. Salmon Fish Cakes

Preparing time: 25 minutes

Serves: 8

Ingredients:

- 2 large eggs
- 4 oz. of sliced smoked salmon
- ½ tbsp. of butter
- 2 tbsp. of fresh chives
- Salt and pepper
- Jar of ready-made Hollandaise sauce

Directions:

1. Boil the eggs for 10 to 12 minutes. They need to be hard boiled.
2. Dice the salmon finely while the eggs are cooking.
3. Heat the butter under a high heat. Put half the salmon in to crisp it up, then set aside.
4. Run the eggs under cold water and peel.

5. Mash the eggs using a fork until they are broken up into fine pieces.
6. Take the raw salmon and half of the chives and mix with the egg and 2 to 3 tbsp. of Hollandaise sauce.
7. Split the mixture into four lumps and form into rough balls.
8. Mix the crispy salmon and remaining chives together and dip the egg balls into them until fully coated.

Nutritional Information Per Serving
(Calories: 295 | Total Fat: 23g | Net Carbs: 1g | Protein 18g | Fiber: 7.3g)

38. Bistro Steak Salad with Horseradish Dressing

Preparing time: 35 minutes

Serves: 2

Ingredients:

- 1 (12 oz.) rib-eye steak
- ¼ tsp. of both salt and pepper
- 1 small red onion
- 1 bag romaine salad greens
- 4 slices of uncured bacon
- ½ cup of sliced radishes

Dressing:

- 2 tbsp. prepared horseradish
- ¼ cup of mayonnaise
- Pepper and salt

Directions:

1. Thinly slice the onion and radishes.
2. Place parchment paper on a baking tin. Set the oven temperature to 350°F. Arrange the bacon in a single layer in the pan. Bake for 15 minutes. Drain and break into small pieces.

3. Pat the steak with paper towels. Season with the pepper and salt. Grill for four minutes and flip. Continue cooking another 12-15 minutes (medium heat for approximately 12 minutes or internal temperature of 155°F).

4. Let it cool down five minutes, and slice against the grain into small slices.

5. Prepare the dressing and enjoy.

Nutritional Information Per Serving (Calories: 167 | Total Fat: 59.4g | Net Carbs: 6.2g | Protein: 41.4g)

39. Low-Carb Mayonnaise for the Horseradish Dressing

Preparing time: 25 minutes

Serves: 8

Ingredients:

- 1 egg yolk
- 1-2 tsp. white vinegar/lemon juice
- 1 tbsp. Dijon mustard
- 1 cup light olive oil

Directions:

1. Ahead of time, take out the egg and mustard to become room temperature.
2. Mix the mustard and egg. Slowly, pour the oil until the mixture thickens.
3. Pour in the lemon juice/vinegar. Stir well. Add a pinch of salt and pepper for additional flavoring.

Nutritional Information Per Serving **(Calories: 217 | Total Fat: 59.4g | Net Carbs: 6.2g | Protein: 41.4 g | Fiber: 7.3g)**

40. Caprese Salad

Preparing time: 45 minutes

Serves: 5

Ingredients:

- 3 cups of grape tomatoes
- 4 peeled garlic cloves
- 2 tbsp. avocado oil
- 10 pearl-sized mozzarella balls
- 4 cups baby spinach leaves
- ¼ cup fresh basil leaves
- 1 tbsp. of each: Brine reserved from the cheese and Pesto

Directions:

1. Use aluminum foil to cover a baking tray. Pre-heat the oven to 400°F. Arrange the cloves and tomatoes on the baking pan and drizzle with the oil.
2. Bake 20-30 minutes until the tops are slightly browned.
3. Drain the liquid (saving one tablespoon) from the mozzarella. Mix the pesto with the brine.
4. Arrange the spinach in a large serving bowl. Transfer the tomatoes to the dish

along with the roasted garlic. Drizzle with the pesto sauce.

5. Garnish with the mozzarella balls, and freshly torn basil leaves.

Nutritional Information Per Serving (Calories: 190.75 | Total Fat: 63.49g | Net Carbs: 4.58g | Protein: 7.71 g)

41. Egg Salad Stuffed Avocado

Preparing time: 20 minutes

Serves: 5

Ingredients:

- 6 large hard boiled eggs
- 3 celery ribs
- ⅓ medium red onion
- 4 tbsp. mayonnaise
- 2 tbsp. fresh lime juice
- 2 tsp. brown mustard
- Pepper and salt, to taste
- ½ tsp. cumin
- 1 tsp. hot sauce
- 3 medium avocados

Directions:

1. Begin by chopping the onions, celery and eggs. Discard the pit and slice the avocado in half.

2. Combine with all of the other fixings, except for the avocado.

3. Scoop the salad into the avocado and serve!

Nutritional Information Per Serving **(Calories: 280.57 | Total Fat: 24.83g | Net Carbs: 3.03g | Protein: 8.32g | Fiber: 7.3g)**

42. Thai Pork Salad

Preparing time: 25 minutes

Serves: 5

Ingredients:

- 2 cup romaine lettuce
- 10 oz. pulled pork
- ¼ medium chopped red bell pepper
- ¼ cup chopped cilantro

Sauce:

- 2 tbsp. of tomato paste
- 2 tbsp. chopped cilantro
- Juice & zest of 1 lime
- 2 tbsp. (+) 2 tsp. soy sauce
- 1 tsp. of red curry paste
- 1 tsp. of five spice
- 1 tsp. of fish sauce
- ¼ tsp. red pepper flakes
- 1 tbsp. (+) 1 tsp. rice wine vinegar
- ½ tsp. mango extract
- 10 drops liquid stevia

Directions:

1. Zest half of the lime and chop the cilantro.

2. Mix all of the sauce fixings.

3. Blend the barbecue sauce components and set aside.

4. Pull the pork apart and make the salad.

5. Pour a glaze over the pork with a bit of the sauce.

Nutritional Information Per Serving (Calories: 216 | Total Fat: 32.6g | Net Carbs: 5.2g | Protein: 29.2g | Fiber: 7.3g)

43. Vegetarian Club Salad

Preparing time: 25 minutes

Serves: 5

Ingredients:

- 2 tbsp. mayonnaise
- 2 tbsp. sour cream
- ½ tsp. of onion powder
- ½ tsp. garlic powder
- 1 tbsp. milk
- 1 tsp. dried parsley
- 3 large hard boiled eggs
- 4 oz. cheddar cheese
- ½ cup cherry tomatoes
- 1 cup diced cucumber
- 3 cups torn romaine lettuce
- 1 tbsp. Dijon mustard

Directions:

1. Slice the hard boiled eggs and cube the cheese. Cut the tomatoes into halves and dice the cucumber.

2. Prepare the dressing (dried herbs, mayo and sour cream) mixing well.

3. Add one tablespoon of milk to the mixture - and another if it's too thick.

4. Layer the salad with the vegetables, cheese and egg slices. Scoop a spoonful of mustard in the center along with a drizzle of dressing.

5. Toss and enjoy!

Nutritional Information Per Serving (Calories: 329.67| Total Fat: 26.32g | Net Carbs: 4.83g | Protein: 16.82g | Fiber: 7.3g)

44. Cumin Spiced Beef Wraps

Preparing time: 25 minutes

Serves: 5

Ingredients:

- 1-2 tbsp. of coconut oil
- ¼ onion, diced
- ⅔ lb. ground beef
- 2 tbsp. of chopped cilantro
- 1 diced red bell pepper
- 1 tsp. of minced ginger
- 2 tsp. of cumin
- 4 minced garlic cloves
- Pepper and salt, to your liking
- 8 large cabbage leaves

Directions:

1. Warm up a frying pan and pour in the oil. Sauté the peppers, onions, and ground beef using medium heat. When done, add the pepper, salt, cumin, ginger, cilantro and garlic.

2. Fill a large pot with water (¾ full) and wait for it to boil. Cook each leaf for 20 seconds, plunge it in cold water and drain before placing it on your serving dish.

3. Scoop the mixture onto each leaf, fold and enjoy.

Nutritional Values Per Serving (Calories: 375 | Total Fat: 26g | Net Carbs: 4g | Protein: 30g | Fiber: 7.3g)

45. Balsamic Beef Pot Roast

Preparing time: 35 minutes

Serves: 5

Ingredients:

- 1 boneless (approx. 3 lb.) chuck roast
- 1 tsp. of garlic powder
- 1 tsp. of black ground pepper
- 1 tbsp. kosher salt
- ¼ cup of balsamic vinegar
- ½ cup of chopped onion
- 2 cups of water
- ¼ tsp. of xanthan gum
- Freshly chopped parsley, for garnish

Directions:

1. Combine the salt, garlic powder and pepper and rub the chuck roast with the combined fixings.
2. Use a heavy skillet to sear the roast. Add the vinegar and deglaze the pan as you continue cooking for one more minute.

3. Toss the onion into a pot with the (two cups) boiling water along with the roast. Cover with a top and simmer for three to four hours on a low setting.

4. Take the meat from the pot and add to a cutting surface. Shred into chunks and remove any fat or bones.

5. Add the xanthan gum to the broth and whisk.

6. Place the roast meat back in the pan to warm up.

7. Serve with a favorite side dish.

Nutritional Information Per Serving (**Calories: 393 | Total Fat: 28g | Net Carbs: 3g | Protein: 30g | Fiber: 7.3g)**

46. Cheeseburger Calzone

Preparing time: 25 minutes

Serves: 5

Ingredients:

- ½ yellow onion, diced
- 1 ½ lb. ground beef, lean
- 4 thick-cut bacon strips
- 4 dill pickle spears
- 8 oz. cream cheese, divided
- 1 egg
- ½ cup mayonnaise
- 1 cup of shredded cheddar cheese
- 1 cup of almond flour
- 1 cup of shredded mozzarella cheese

Directions:

1. Pre-heat the oven to 425°F. Prepare a cookie tin with parchment paper.
2. Chop the pickles into spears. Set aside for now.
3. Prepare the Crust: Combine ½ of the cream cheese and the mozzarella cheese. Microwave 35 seconds. When it melts, add the egg and almond flour to make the dough. Set aside.
4. Cook the beef on the stove using medium heat.

5. Cook the bacon (microwave for five minutes or stovetop). When cool, break into bits.
6. Dice the onion and add to the beef and cook until softened. Toss in the bacon, cheddar cheese, pickle bits, the rest of the cream cheese and mayonnaise. Stir well.
7. Roll the dough onto the prepared baking tin. Scoop the mixture into the center. Fold the ends and side to make the calzone.
8. Bake until browned or about 15 minutes. Let it rest for 10 minutes before slicing.

Nutritional Information Per Serving (Calories: 187 | Total Fat: 47g | Net Carbs: 3g | Protein: 34g | Fiber: 7.3g)

47. Vegetarian Keto Burger on a Bun

Preparing time: 35 minutes

Serves: 5

Ingredients:

- 1-2 tbsp. freshly chopped basil – 1 tsp. dried
- 2 medium-large flat mushrooms
- 1 tbsp. of coconut oil/ghee
- 1 tbsp. freshly chopped oregano – ½ tsp. dried
- 1 crushed garlic clove
- ¼ tsp. salt
- Black pepper
- 2 large organic eggs
- 2 slices cheddar/gouda cheese
- 2 tbsp. mayonnaise
- 2 keto buns – see recipe below

Directions:

1. Prepare the mushrooms for marinating by seasoning with crushed garlic, pepper, salt, ghee (melted) and fresh herbs. Save a small amount for frying the eggs. Marinate for about one hour at room temperature.
2. Arrange the mushrooms in the pan with the top side facing upwards. Cook for about five minutes on the med-high

setting. Flip and continue cooking for another five minutes.

3. Remove the pan from the burner and flip the mushrooms over and add the cheese. When it is time to serve, put them under the broiler for a minute or so to melt the cheese.
4. With the remainder of the ghee, fry the eggs leaving the yolk runny. Remove from the heat.
5. Slice the buns and add them to the grill, cooking until crisp for about two to three minutes.
6. To assemble, add one tablespoon of mayonnaise to each bun and top them off with the mushroom, egg, tomato and lettuce.

Nutritional Information Per Serving (Calories: 211 | Total Fat: 55.1g | Net Carbs: 8.7g | Protein: 23.7g | Fiber: 7.3g)

48. Barbecue Pulled Chicken in the Slow Cooker

Preparing time: 35 minutes

Serves: 5

Ingredients:

- 3 lb. chicken thighs
- 1 tsp. of cumin
- 1 tsp. of smoked paprika
- 1 tsp. of onion powder
- ¼ tsp. of pepper
- ¾ tsp. salt - divided
- 1 tsp. of maple extract
- ¼ cup of apple cider vinegar
- 1 cup of sugar-free ketchup
- ½ cup of water
- ½ tsp. of clear liquid stevia
- 1 tbsp. of unsweetened cocoa powder
- ¼ tsp. of cumin

Directions:

1. Remove all of the bones and chicken and arrange the chicken on a baking sheet. Combine the salt, pepper, cumin,

onion powder, and paprika together. Rub it over the chicken.

2. Pour the ketchup, vinegar, and water into the slow cooker. Stir, and add the rest of the fixings. Lastly, add the chicken.

3. Close the lid and cook four hours on high or eight hours on low.

4. Enjoy over some rice (add the carbs).

Nutritional Information Per Serving: **Calories: 219| Fat: 7.2 g| Carbohydrates: 4.3 g| Protein: 33.8 g Fiber: 7.3g**

49. Beef Patties

Preparing time: 20 minutes

Serves: 6

Ingredients:

- ½ cup bread crumbs
- 1 egg
- Salt and ground black pepper, to taste
- 1½ pounds ground beef
- 10 ounces canned onion soup
- 1 tablespoon coconut flour
- ¼ cup ketchup
- 3 teaspoons Worcestershire sauce
- ½ teaspoon dry mustard
- ¼ cup water

1. In a bowl, mix ⅓ cup of the onion soup with the beef, salt, pepper, egg, and bread crumbs, and stir well.

2. Heat up a pan over medium-high heat, shape 6 patties from the beef mixture, place them into the pan, and brown on both sides.

3. In a bowl, mix the rest of the soup with the coconut flour, water, dry mustard,

Worcestershire sauce, and ketchup, and stir well.

4. Pour this over the beef patties, cover pan, and cook for 20 minutes stirring from time to time.

5. Divide on plates and serve.

Nutritional Information Per Serving:
Calories - 332, Fat – 18g, Fiber – 1g, Carbs – 7g, Protein – 25g

50. Ground Beef Bacon Cheeseburger Casserole

Preparing time: 25 minutes

Serves: 5

Ingredients:

- 3 bacon slices
- 1 lb. (80/20) ground beef
- ½ cup of almond flour
- 2 ½ cups of riced cauliflower (265g)
- ½ tsp. of onion powder
- ½ tsp. of garlic powder
- 1 tbsp. Psyllium husk powder
- 2 tbsp. of ketchup – reduced-sugar
- 2 tbsp. of mayonnaise
- 1 tbsp. Dijon mustard
- 3 large eggs
- Pepper and salt, to taste
- 4 oz. cheddar cheese, divided

Directions:

1. Pre-heat the oven setting to 350°F.
2. Toss in the bacon and ground beef. Pulse until it's a bit pasty and crumbly. Cook the mixture over the medium-high setting on the stove.

3. Combine all of the components in a mixing dish and add ½ of the cheese.

4. Press into a parchment paper-lined pan and top it off with the rest of the cheese.

5. Bake 25-30 minutes on the top oven rack. Let it cool about 5 to 10 minutes before serving.

Nutritional Information Per Serving (Calories: 132 | Total Fats: 35.5g | Net Carbs: 3.6g | Protein: 32.2 g | Fiber: 7.3g)

51. BBQ & Bacon Cheeseburger Waffles

Preparing time: 35 minutes
Serves: 5
Ingredients:

Waffles

- 1 ½ oz. cheddar cheese
- 1 cup of cauliflower crumbles
- 2 large eggs
- ¼ tsp. of onion powder
- ¼ tsp. of garlic powder
- 3 tbsp. of grated parmesan cheese
- 4 tbsp. of almond flour
- Pepper and salt, to taste

Topping

- 4 oz. of (70/30) ground beef
- 4 tbsp. of BBQ sauce, sugar-free
- 4 bacon slices
- 1 ½ oz. cheddar cheese
- Salt and pepper, to taste

Directions:

1. Shred all of the cheese, and divide into two bowls.

2. Combine the eggs, ½ of the cheddar cheese, spices, flour and parmesan cheese.
3. Prepare the bacon on the stove using the medium-high setting. When done, toss in the beef and cook until done (set aside for Step 5).
4. Add the excess of grease into the waffle mixture. Make a thick paste with the blender.
5. Add ½ of the mix into the waffle iron and repeat with the remainder of the mix.
6. For each waffle, add ½ of the beef, and ½ of the cheese on top. Broil for 1 to 2 minutes until the cheese melts.

Nutritional Information Per Serving (Calories: 123.25 | Total Fats: 33.94g | Net Carbs: 4.35g| Protein: 18.8g | Fiber: 7.3g)

52. Thai Beef

Preparing time: 20 minutes

Serves: 6

Ingredients:

- 1 cup beef stock
- 4 tablespoons peanut butter
- ¼ teaspoon garlic powder
- ¼ teaspoon onion powder
- 1 tablespoon coconut aminos
- 1½ teaspoons lemon pepper
- 1 pound beef steak, cut into strips
- Salt and ground black pepper, to taste
- 1 green bell pepper, seeded and chopped
- 3 green onions, chopped

Directions:

In a bowl, mix the peanut butter with the stock, aminos, and lemon pepper, stir well, and set aside. Heat up a pan over medium-high heat, add the beef, season with salt, pepper, onion, and garlic powder, and cook for 7 minutes. Add the green pepper, stir, and cook for 3 minutes. Add the peanut sauce and green onions, stir, cook for 1 minute, divide on plates, and serve.

Nutritional Information Per Serving: **(Calories: 224 | Total Fat : 15g | Fiber : 1g | Carbs : 3g | Protein : 19g)**

53. Cumin Spiced Beef Wraps

Preparing time: 20 minutes
Serves: 5

Ingredients:

- 1-2 tbsp. of coconut oil
- ¼ onion – diced
- ⅔ lb. ground beef
- 2 tsp. of cumin
- 4 minced garlic cloves
- Pepper and salt, to taste
- 8 large cabbage leaves

Directions:

1. Warm up a frying pan and pour in the oil. Sauté the peppers, onions and ground beef using medium-heat.

2. When done, add the pepper, salt, cumin, ginger, cilantro and garlic.

3. Fill a large pot with water (¾ full) and wait for it to boil. Cook each leaf for 20 seconds, plunge it in cold water and drain before placing it on your serving dish.

4. Scoop the mixture onto each leaf, fold and enjoy.

Nutritional Information Per Serving (Calories: 375 | Total Fats: 26g | Net Carbs: 4g | Protein: 30 g | Fiber: 7.3g)

54. Portobello Bun Cheeseburgers

Preparing time: 35 minutes

Serves: 5

Ingredients:

- 1 tbsp. of Worcestershire sauce
- 1 lb. (80/20) ground beef
- 1 tsp. of Pink Himalayan salt
- 1 tsp. of ground black pepper
- 1 tbsp. of avocado oil
- 6 slices sharp cheddar cheese
- 6 Portobello mushroom caps

Directions:

1. Remove the stem, rinse and dab dry the mushrooms.
2. Combine the salt, pepper, beef and Worcestershire sauce in a mixing container. Form into patties.

3. Transfer the mushrooms to a bowl and using the same pan - cook the patties 4 minutes, flip and cook another 5 minutes until done.

4. Add the cheese to the burgers and cover for 1 minute to melt the cheese.

5. Add one of the mushroom caps to the burgers along with the desired garnishes and serve.

Nutritional Information Per Serving (Calories: 336 | Total Fats: 22.8g | Net Carbs: 4g | Protein: 29.1g | Fiber: 7.3g)

55. BBQ Pulled Beef Sando – Slow Cooker

Preparing time: 25 minutes

Serves: 5

Ingredients:

- 3 lbs. boneless chuck roast
- 2 tsp. of garlic powder
- 2 tsp. Pink Himalayan salt
- 1 tsp. of black pepper
- 1 tsp. of onion powder
- 1 tbsp. of smoked paprika
- ¼ cup of apple cider vinegar
- 2 tbsp. of tomato paste
- 2 tbsp. of coconut aminos
- ½ cup of bone broth
- ¼ cup of melted butter

Directions:

1. Remove all of the fat from the beef and cut it half to fit in the cooker.
2. Rub the beef and arrange the pieces in the pot.

3. In another container, melt the butter and whisk in the amino, vinegar and tomato paste. Pour the mixture over the roast and add the bone broth.

4. Set on the low setting to cook for 10-12 hours.

5. Once it's done, raise the heat to high and let the sauce thicken. Shred the beef and add it back and toss.

Nutritional Information Per Serving (Calories: 184 | Total Fats: 5.1g | Net Carbs: 3.6g | Protein: 5.1g | Fiber: 7.3g)

56. Bone Broth for the BBQ

Preparing time: 40 minutes

Serves: 5

Ingredients:

- Purified water
- 1 tbsp. vinegar, white or apple cider
- Bones from grass-fed beef

Directions:

1. Pour in the vinegar.
2. Set the pot on the low setting for 6 hours (minimum).
3. *Note:* Beef can simmer 48 hours/chicken 24 hours.
4. Empty the broth through a sieve into a container. Remove the bones with a pair of tongs.
5. You can use it for up to one week or freeze for another recipe later.

Nutritional Information Per Serving (Calories: 154 | Total Fats: 39.4g | Net Carb: 2.1g| Protein: 29.4g)

57. Beef Wellington

Preparing time: 25 minutes

Serves: 5

Ingredients:

- 2 (4 lb. or 13g) tenderloin steaks
- 1 tbsp. of butter
- Pepper and salt, to taste
- 1 cup of shredded mozzarella cheese
- ½ cup of almond flour
- 4 tbsp. of liver pâté

Directions:

1. Pre-heat the oven temperature to 400°F.
2. Salt and pepper the steaks and melt the butter on the medium-high heat.
3. Place the meat in the pan when it's hot and sear. Flip them over every 2 or 3 minutes. Let them cool.
4. Warm up the cheese in a microwave about 1 minute. Arrange the dough in between two pieces of parchment paper. Use a rolling pin (or wine bottle) to flatten the dough. Slice it so you can form a circular ball.

5. Add one tablespoon of the pâté onto the dough. (It needs to be large enough to fit around the meat and the pâté.)

6. Bake for about 20 to 30 minutes and enjoy.

Nutritional Information Per Serving (Calories: 307.5| Total Fats: 22.66g | Net Carbs: 2.31g | Protein: 23.6g | Fiber: 7.3g)

58. Mississippi Chuck Roast in the Slow Cooker

Preparing time: 15 minutes

Serves: 4

Ingredients:

- 1 (3.8 lbs.) beef chuck roast
- 1 jar (16 oz.) deli-sliced pepperoncini
- 1 tbsp. of dried dill
- 1 tbsp. of garlic powder
- 1 tbsp. of dried parsley
- 1 tbsp. of dried chives
- 1 tbsp. of onion powder
- ½ tsp. of salt
- ¼ tsp. of black pepper
- 2 tbsp. of Better than Bouillon

Directions:

1. Drain and reserve the brine in the pepperoncini.
2. Place the cooker on the high setting and add to the roast along with the pepperoncini.

3. Stir in the spices and the bouillon paste. Top it off with the stick of butter.

4. Cook on the high setting for 8 to 10 hours. No need to stir.

5. When the roast is done (falling apart), shred it with a fork and serve.

Nutritional Information Per Serving (Calories: 123.22 | Total Fats: 31.64g | Net Carbs: 3.13g | Protein: 33.21 g | Fiber: 7.3g)

59. Nacho Steak – Skillet Style

Preparing time: 45 minutes

Serves: 4

Ingredients:

- 1 tbsp. of butter
- 8 oz. beef round tip steak
- ⅓ cup of melted refined coconut oil
- ½ tsp. of turmeric
- 1 tsp. of chili powder
- 1 ½ lbs. of cauliflower
- 1 oz. of cheddar cheese
- 1 oz. monterey jack cheese

Possible Garnishes:

- 1 oz. of canned jalapeno slices
- ⅓ cup of sour cream
- Avocado – Approx. 5 oz.

Directions:

1. Pre-heat the oven temperature to 400°F.
2. Prepare the cauliflower into chip-like shapes.
3. Combine the turmeric, chili powder and coconut oil in a mixing dish.
4. Over medium-high heat in a cast iron skillet, add the butter. Cook until both

sides are done, flipping just once. Let it rest for 5 to 10 minutes. Thinly slice the steak, and sprinkle with some pepper and salt.

5. Transfer the florets when they have finished cooking into the skillet and add the steak strips. Top it off with the cheese and bake 5 to 10 more minutes.

6. Serve with your favorite garnish.

Nutritional Information Per Serving (Calories: 385.4 | Total Fats: 30.67g | Net Carbs: 5.9g | Protein: 18.87 g | Fiber: 7.3g)

60. Steak-Lovers Slow-Cooked Chili in the Slow Cooker

Preparing time: 25 minutes

Serves: 4

Ingredients:

- 1 cup of beef or chicken stock
- ½ cup of sliced leeks
- 2 ½ lbs. (1-inch cubes) steak
- 2 cup of whole tomatoes (canned with juices)

Optional Toppings:

- 1 tsp. fresh chopped cilantro
- 2 tbsp. sour cream
- ¼ cup of shredded cheddar cheese
- ½ avocado – sliced or cubed

Directions:

1. Toss all of the fixings into the cooker - except the toppings.

2. Use the cooker's high setting for about 6 hours.

3. Serve, add the toppings and enjoy.

Nutritional Information Per Serving (Calories: 321 | Total Fats: 26.0g | Net Carbs: 3.3g | Protein: 38.4 g| Fiber: 7.3g)

Chapter 10: Dinner Recipes

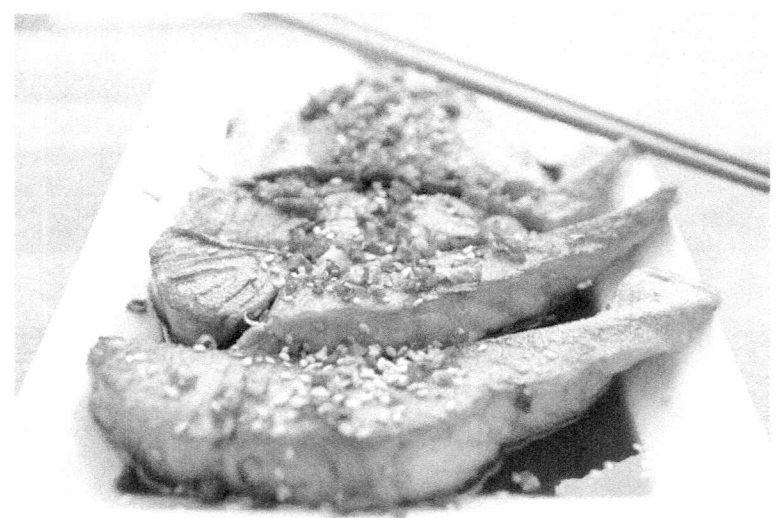

61. Chicken and Asparagus Pan Dinner

Preparing time: 35 minutes

Serves: 4

Ingredients:

- 4 lbs. chicken breasts
- 1 tbsp. of avocado oil
- 1 lb. trimmed asparagus
- 4 sun-dried tomatoes
- 4 pieces of thick-cut bacon
- 1 tsp. salt
- ¼ tsp. pepper
- 8 slices of provolone cheese

Directions:

1. Prepare the chicken into 8 thin pieces. Chop the bacon and tomatoes into 1-inch pieces.
2. Pre-heat the oven temperature to 400°F.
3. Add the oil to the baking pan along with the chicken and asparagus. Top it off with the tomatoes and bacon. Sprinkle some pepper and salt for seasoning.

4. Bake until the chicken reaches 160°F internally or about 25 minutes.

5. Toss in the asparagus and cheese. Garnish with some bacon and tomatoes. Bake another 3 to 4 minutes until the cheese has melted.

Nutritional Information Per Serving (Calories: 324| Total Fats: 18.2g | Net Carbs: 4g | Protein: 63g | Fiber: 7.3g)

62. Chicken Kiev

Preparing time: 45 minutes
Serves: 4

Ingredients:

- 2 (6 oz.) breasts of chicken
- 2 cloves of garlic
- 4 tbsp. butter
- 1 stalk green onion
- Parsley
- Tarragon
- Pepper and salt, to taste
- 1 oz. pork rinds
- ¼ cup of coconut flour
- 1 egg

Directions:

1. Set the oven temperature to 350°F.
2. Use a tenderizing hammer to pound the chicken until they are approximately ½-inch to 1-inch thick. Flavor it with the tarragon, pepper, salt and parsley.
3. Add chopped bits of butter, garlic and green onion evenly to the pieces of chicken. Close with toothpicks.

4. Crush the pork rinds for the crumbs (NutriBullet for a few seconds works great.)

5. Make dredging dishes; one each for flour, a beaten egg and the pork rind crumbs.

6. Cover the chicken with the flour, egg, then the rinds. Close them tightly with a toothpick. Let the fixings chill in the fridge for about ½ hour.

7. Fry the breasts until browned on all sides in a lightly oiled pan.

8. Transfer and arrange them in a baking dish.

9. Bake for approximately 20 minutes. Baste with any leftover butter.

10. Serve on a bed of lettuce.

Nutritional Information Per Serving (Calories: 134 | Total Fats: 33g | Net Carbs: 4g | Protein: 50g | Fiber: 7.3g)

63. Chicken Pad Thai

Preparing time: 25 minutes
Serves: 4
Ingredients:

- ⅛ tsp. of freshly ground black pepper
- ⅛ tsp. of garlic powder
- ⅛ tsp. of sea salt
- ⅛ tsp. of ground ginger
- 2 lbs. chicken tenders
- 2 tbsp. of peanut oil
- 3 tbsp. of peanut butter
- 3 large eggs, lightly beaten
- ⅓ cup of organic chicken broth
- 1 tbsp. of rice vinegar
- 2 tbsp. of tamari
- 2 minced garlic cloves
- ½ cup of chopped scallion
- 1 tsp. of red pepper flakes
- 4 spiralized zucchini
- ½ cup of bean sprouts

Garnish:

- ½ cup of crushed peanuts
- 1 lime - wedges

Directions:

1. Combine the pepper, salt, garlic powder and ginger. Toss the chicken in the spices.
2. Add the tenders and cook about 3 minutes (turning once). Slice into ¼-inch slices and set aside for now.
3. Scramble the eggs about 1 minute and set aside.
4. Pour in the broth, tamari, peanut butter, scallion, vinegar, red pepper flakes and garlic. Cook for 3 minutes – stir well.
5. Blend in the zucchini noodles, chicken slices, sprouts and eggs into the pan. Toss and cook about 1 minute.

Nutritional Information Per Serving (Calories: 219 | Total Fats: 34g | Net Carbs: 8g | Protein: 90g | Fiber: 7.3g)

64. Chicken Parmesan

Preparing time: 25 minutes

Serves: 4

Ingredients:

- 1 lb. breasts of chicken
- 2 tbsp. of parmesan cheese
- 1 oz. pork rinds
- 1 egg
- ½ cup of marinara sauce
- ½ cup of shredded mozzarella

Possible Garnish:

- Garlic powder
- Salt and pepper
- Oregano

Directions:

1. Program the oven temperature to 350°F.
2. Use a food processor to crush the pork rinds and parmesan cheese. Add them to a bowl.
3. Pound the chicken breasts until they are ½-inch thick. Beat the egg and dip the

chicken in for an egg wash. Dip the chicken into the crumbs.

4. Dump the marinara sauce over each portion. Garnish with the mozzarella and bake for 15 minutes.

5. Enjoy with a bed of spinach.

Nutritional Information Per Serving (Calories: 167 | Total Fats: 32g | Net Carbs: 3g | Protein: 74g | Fiber: 7.3g)

65. Chicken Smothered in Creamy Onion Sauce

Preparing time: 35 minutes

Serves: 4

Ingredients:

- 1 whole green/spring onion
- 2 tbsp. or 1 oz. butter
- 4 chicken breast halves (skinless—boneless / 6 oz. approx.)
- 8 oz. sour cream
- ½ tsp. sea salt

Directions:

1. Use the medium-high setting to melt the butter in a skillet. Reduce the setting to medium-low. Arrange the chicken with the butter. Cover and cook about 10 additional minutes.

2. Chop the onion using the white and green sections.

3. Flip the breasts. Cover and simmer another 8 or 9 minutes or until thoroughly done.

4. Combine the onion and cook an additional 1 or 2 minutes.

5. Take it off the burner, and blend in the sour cream and salt.

6. Wait for about 5 minutes. Mix well and serve.

Nutritional Information Per Serving (Calories: 178 | Total Fats: 26g | Net Carbs: 3.3g | Protein: 38.4g | Fiber: 7.3g)

66. Chicken Stuffed Avocado—Cajun Style

Preparing time: 25 minutes

Serves: 4

Ingredients:

- 1 ½ cup of cooked chicken (7.4 oz.)
- 1 large or 2 medium avocados (10.6 oz.)
- 2 tbsp. of cream cheese/sour cream
- 2 tbsp. of lemon juice (fresh)
- ¼ cup of mayonnaise
- ¼ tsp. of cayenne pepper
- ¼ tsp. of salt
- ½ tsp. of onion powder
- ½ tsp. of garlic powder
- 1 tsp. of paprika
- 1 tsp. of dried thyme

Directions:

1. Shred the chicken into small pieces.
2. Blend all the ingredients—saving the salt and lemon juice until last.

3. Leave ½ to 1-inch of the avocado flesh—scoop the middle. Remove the pits.

4. Cut the center/scooped pieces of avocado into small pieces and fill each of the halves with the mixture of chicken.

Nutritional Information Per Serving (Calories: 189 | Total Fats: 50.6g | Net Carbs: 5.4g| Protein: 34.5g | Fiber: 7.3g)

67. Coconut Curry Chicken Tenders

Preparing time: 45 minutes
Serves: 4

Ingredients:

Tenders:
- 1 large egg
- 1 pkg. chicken thighs (24 oz./ 5 thighs), deboned with skin
- ½ cup of crumbled pork rinds (1 ½ oz.)
- Unsweetened shredded coconut
- ½ tsp. of coriander
- 2 tsp. of curry powder
- ¼ tsp. of onion powder
- ¼ tsp. of garlic powder
- Pepper and salt, to taste

Sweet and Spicy Mango Dipping Sauce:
- ¼ cup of sour cream
- ¼ cup of mayonnaise
- 1 ½ tsp. of mango extract
- 2 tbsp. of sugar-free ketchup
- ¼ tsp. of cayenne pepper
- ½ tsp. of ground ginger and ½ tsp. of garlic powder
- Red pepper flakes
- 7 drops liquid stevia

Directions:

1. Pre-heat the oven to 400°F.
2. Whisk the eggs and debone the thighs. Slice them into strips (skins on).
3. Add the spices, coconut and pork rinds to a Ziploc-type bag. Add the chicken, shake and place on a wire rack. Flip them over and continue baking for another 20 minutes.
4. Combine the sauce components and stir well.
5. Serve with your tasty chicken tenders

Nutritional Information Per Serving
(Calories: **180** | Total Fats: 39.4g | Net Carbs: 2.1g | Protein: 29.4g | Fiber: 7.3g)

68. Beef Pot Roast

Preparing time: 45 minutes

Serves: 4

Ingredients:

- 3½ pounds beef roast
- 4 oz. mushrooms, sliced
- 12 oz. beef stock
- 1 oz. onion soup mix
- ½ cup Italian dressing

Directions:

1. Pre-heat the oven to 300°F.
2. In a bowl, mix the stock with the onion soup mixture and Italian dressing, and stir.
3. Put the beef roast in a pan, add the mushrooms, stock mixture, cover with aluminum foil, place in an o
4. Let the roast to cool, slice, and serve with the gravy on top.

Nutritional Information Per Serving (Calories: 700 | Total Fats: 56g | Net Carbs: 10g | Fiber: 2g | Protein - 70 g)

69. Italian Chicken and Cauliflower Casserole

Preparing time: 35 minutes

Serves: 4

Ingredients:

- 1 pkg. (20 oz.) chicken breast
- 1 tbsp. of olive oil
- 2 ½ oz. mushrooms
- 2 cups of riced cauliflower
- ¼ cup of mayonnaise
- ¼ cup of heavy cream
- ½ cup of low-carb vodka sauce
- 1 cup of shredded mozzarella cheese
- 2 tbsp. of parmesan cheese
- 1 oz. pork rinds
- Salt and pepper
- Oregano
- Garlic powder

Directions:

1. Pre-heat the oven to 375°F.

2. Rice the cauliflower for 10-15 minutes with one cup of boiling chicken broth (the broth should completely evaporate). Add the cream and cook for 5 minutes.

3. Prepare the chicken and shred it into bite-sized chunks. Combine with the mushrooms and mayonnaise. Add the vodka sauce and mix well.

4. Empty the fixings into a rectangular baking dish. Garnish with the cheeses and pork rinds.

5. Bake 20 minutes, topping the baked mixture off with fresh basil.

Nutritional Information Per Serving (Calories: 300 | Total Fats: 21g | Net Carbs: 2.5g |Protein: 29g | Fiber: 7.3g

70. Italian Chicken & Egg Bake

Preparing time: 25 minutes

Serves: 4

Ingredients:

- 10 large eggs
- 2 tsp. garlic and herb seasoning
- 3 tbsp. of mustard
- ½ cup of tomato sauce
- ½ cup of heavy whipping cream
- 2 cups cooked chicken breasts, diced
- 1 pkg. (12.oz.) of frozen broccoli florets
- 1 tsp. of parsley flakes

Directions:

1. Pre-heat the oven temperature to 350°F. Grease a large baking pan or casserole dish.

2. Whisk the eggs and add the garlic, mustard, seasoning and whipping cream. Blend well and mix in the tomato sauce, stirring to remove the lumps. Toss in the florets and chicken.

3. Bake approximately 30-40 minutes. The top will look like a crust.

4. Top it off with some extra sharp cheese, pepper jack or mozzarella. Enjoy!

Nutritional Information Per Serving (**Calories:** 307 | Total Fats: 12.13g | Net Carbs: 2.35g |Protein: 13.3 g | Fiber: 7.3g)

71. Kung Pao Chicken

Preparing time: 25 minutes

Serves: 4

Ingredients:

- 2 med. (bone-in) chicken thighs with skins
- 1 tsp. of ground ginger
- 2 large spring onions
- ½ med. green pepper
- ¼ cup peanuts
- Pepper and salt, to taste
- 4 red Bird's Eye Chilis, deseeded

Sauce:

- 2 tsp. of rice wine vinegar, 2 tbsp. of chili garlic paste
- 2 tsp. of sesame oil, 1 tbsp. of soy sauce
- Reduced-sugar ketchup
- 10 drops liquid stevia and ½ tsp. of maple extract

Directions:

1. Slice the chicken into bite-sized bits and add in with some ginger, pepper and salt.

2. Prepare a skillet on the medium-high setting. Arrange the chicken in the pan and simmer around 10 minutes.

3. Prepare the veggies and chilies. Make the sauce by combining all of the components – stirring well.

4. When the chicken is browned to your liking; combine all of the ingredients to warm up for a few minutes.

5. Toss in the chopped veggies and peanuts and simmer for 3 to 4 minutes. Add the sauce and let it boil until reduced.

Nutritional Information Per Serving (Calories: 362 | Total Fats: 27.4g | Net Carbs: 3.2g | Protein: 22.3 g | Fiber: 7.3g)

72. Nacho Chicken Casserole

Preparing time: 45 minutes

Serves: 4

Ingredients:

- 4 oz. of cheddar cheese
- 4 oz. of cream cheese
- 3 tbsp. of parmesan cheese
- 1 cup of green chilis and tomatoes
- ¼ cup of sour cream
- 1 med. jalapeno pepper
- 1 pkg. frozen cauliflower
- Pepper and salt, to taste

Directions:

1. Pre-heat the oven to 375°F.
2. Slice the jalapeno into bits and set aside.
3. Chop up and pepper and salt the thighs. Cook in olive oil on medium-high until browned.
4. Blend in the sour cream, cream cheese and ¾ of the cheddar cheese. Stir until melted and combined well.

5. Pour in the tomatoes and chilis. Stir and add it all to a baking dish.

6. Cook the cauliflower in the microwave until done.

7. Blend in the rest of the cheese with the immersion blender until it resembles mashed potatoes. Season as desired.

8. Spread the cauliflower concoction over the casserole and sprinkle with the peppers.

9. Bake approximately 15-20 minutes.

Nutritional Information Per Serving (Calories: 126 | Total Fats: 32.2g | Net Carbs: 4.3g | Protein: 30.8g | Fiber: 7.3g)

73. Tikka Masala Chicken – Slow Cooker

Preparing time: 35 minutes

Serves: 4

Ingredients:

- 1 lb. chicken thighs (no bones or skins)
- 1 ½ lbs. chicken thighs (bone-in)
- 2 tsp. of onion powder
- 2 tbsp. of olive oil
- 1-inch grated ginger root
- 3 minced garlic cloves
- 3 tbsp. of tomato paste
- 5 tsp. of Garam Masala
- 2 tsp. of smoked paprika
- 4 tsp. of kosher salt
- 1 cup of heavy cream
- 1 can (10 oz.) of diced tomatoes
- 1 cup of coconut milk (carton)
- Chopped fresh cilantro
- 1 tsp. Guar gum

Directions:

1. Debone all of the chicken and chop into bite-sized segments.

2. Toss the chicken thighs into the cooker and grate the ginger over the top.

3. Add the rest of the spices along with the tomato paste, diced tomatoes and olive oil; mix well

4. Set the timer for 6 hours on the low setting or 3 hours on high.

5. When done, pour in the rest of the milk, Guar gum, and heavy cream into the pot. Mix into the chicken. Serve with your favorite side.

Nutritional Information Per Serving (Calories: 293 | Total Fats: 41.2g | Net Carbs: 5.8g | Protein: 26 g | Fiber: 7.3g)

74. Pizza Goodies BBQ Meat-Lover's Pizza

Preparing time: 25 minutes

Serves: 4

Ingredients:

- 2 cups (8 oz.) of mozzarella
- 1 tbsp. of psyllium husk powder
- ¾ cup of almond flour
- 3 tbsp. (1 ½ oz.) of cream cheese
- 1 large egg
- ½ tsp. of black pepper
- ½ tsp. of salt
- 1 tbsp. of Italian seasoning

Topping:

- 1 cup (4 oz.) of mozzarella cheese
- BBQ sauce, to taste
- Sliced Kabana/hard salami
- Bacon slices
- Sprinkled oregano (optional)

Directions:

1. Pre-heat the oven to 400°F.

2. Melt the cheese in the microwave until it melts (about 45 seconds). Toss in the cream cheese and egg, mixing well.

3. Blend in the psyllium husk, flour, salt, pepper and Italian seasoning. Make the dough as circular as possible. Bake for 10 minutes.

4. Cover the crust with the toppings and some more cheese.

5. Bake until the cheese is golden, slice and serve.

Nutritional Information Per Serving (Calories: | Total Fats: 27g | Net Carbs: 3.5g | Protein: 18g | Fiber: 7.3g)

75. Beefy Pizza

Preparing time: 35 minutes

Serves: 4

Ingredients:

- 2 large eggs
- 1 pkg. (20 oz.) ground beef
- 28 pepperoni slices
- ½ cup of shredded cheddar cheese
- ½ cup of pizza sauce
- 4 oz. mozzarella cheese

Directions:

1. Combine the eggs, beef and seasonings and place in the skillet to form the crust.
2. Bake until the meat is done or about 15 minutes.
3. Take it out and add the sauce, cheese and toppings. Remove and enjoy!

Nutritional Information Per Serving **(Calories:** 210 | Total Fats: 45g | Net Carbs: 2g | Protein: 44g | Fiber: 7.3g)

76. Chicken Fried Pork Chops

Preparing time: 45 minutes

Serves: 4

Ingredients:

- 1 oz. ground pork rinds
- 1 tbsp. of chopped nuts
- 2 tbsp. of flaxseed meal
- 2 tbsp. of almond flour
- 1 tsp. of salt
- 1 large egg
- 4 tbsp. of fat/oil (your choice)
- 4 medium (bone-out 16 oz. ea.) pork chops

Directions:

1. Combine the flaxseed meal, flour and nut blend.
2. Warm up the oil/fat in a skillet using the medium-high setting.

3. Whisk an egg in a dish and dip the chop. Dip in the rind mixture (Step 1). Coat well and fry for about 4 to 5 minutes for each side. The internal temperature should reach 145°F.

4. Serve and enjoy!

Nutritional Information Per Serving (**Calories: 390 | Total Fats: 20.8g | Net Carbs: 0.8g| Protein: 28.8 g | Fiber: 7.3g**)

77. Parmesan Crusted Pork Chops

Preparing time: 15 minutes

Serves: 4

Ingredients:

- 6 oz. parmesan cheese
- 14 pork chops
- 2 large eggs
- ¾ cup of almond flour
- Pepper and salt, if desired
- Bacon grease, for frying

Directions:

1. Pre-heat the oven to 400°F.
2. Grate the parmesan and mix with the flour and spices.
3. Whisk the eggs in a shallow dish.
4. Dip the chops in the eggs; then the parmesan mixture.

5. Fry in the bacon grease on each side for 1 minute.

6. Arrange on a baking dish in the oven, baking until done.

Nutritional Information Per Serving (**Calories: 354 | Total Fats: 34g | Net Carbs: 3g | Protein: 33g | Fiber: 7.3g**)

78. Skillet Style Sausage and Cabbage Melt

Preparing time: 25 minutes

Serves: 4

Ingredients:

- 4 spicy Italian chicken sausages
- 2 tbsp. of coconut oil
- ½ cup onion
- 1 ½ cups of both green & purple cabbage
- 2 tbsp. of chopped fresh cilantro
- 2 slices (1-oz.) of colby jack cheese

Directions:

1. Discard the sausage casings and rough-chop them. Shred the cabbage and dice the onions.

2. Add the coconut oil, cabbage and onion in a large skillet using the medium-high setting for approximately 8 minutes (the

veggies should be tender). Blend the cheese and cover.

3. Turn the heat off and let it rest 5 minutes as the cheese melts.

4. When it is time to serve—stir gently and add the cilantro.

Nutritional Information Per Serving (Calories: 231 | Total Fats: 14.62g | Net Carbs: 3.52g | Protein: 18.26g | Fiber: 7.3g)

79. Squash and Sausage Casserole

Preparing time: 35 minutes

Serves: 4

Ingredients:

- 1 lb. browned sausage
- 2 large eggs
- 2 med. summer squash
- 1 med. zucchini
- 1 tsp. of salt
- ½ tsp. onion powder or ¼ cup of dried minced onion
- 1 cup of mayonnaise
- 1 pkg. sugar substitute (or stevia)
- ¼ tsp. of pepper
- 1 ½ cups of shredded cheddar cheese, divided
- ¼ of melted butter

Directions:

1. Pre-heat the oven to 350°F.
2. Slice and cook the zucchini and squash.

3. Combine each of the ingredients except for ½ cup of shredded cheese.

4. Dump the ingredients into the lightly greased baking plate. Sprinkle the remainder of cheese on the casserole.

5. Bake until lightly browned for about 30 minutes.

Nutritional Information Per Serving (**Calories: 372 | Total Fats: 34.8g | Net Carbs: 2.0g | Protein: 12.4 g| Fiber: 7.3g**)

80. Chili Lime Cod

Preparing time: 30 minutes

Serves: 4

Ingredients:

- 1 (10-12 oz.) wild-caught cod
- ⅓ cup of coconut flour
- 1 egg
- 1 lime
- ½ tsp. of cayenne pepper
- 1 tsp. of garlic powder
- 1 tsp. of salt
- Crushed red pepper

Directions:

1. Pre-heat the oven to 400°F.
2. In separate dishes, whip the egg and remove any lumps from the flour.
3. Let the fillet soak in the egg dish for 1 minute on each side. Add it to the flour dish, and then add it to a baking sheet.
4. Sprinkle the spices and drizzle the lime juice over the cod.

5. Bake 10 to 12 minutes or when it easily flakes apart.

6. Drizzle with some Sriracha if you wish and enjoy.

Nutritional Information Per Serving **(Calories: 215 | Total Fats: 5g | Net Carbs: 3g | Protein: 37g | Fiber: 7.3g)**

81. Pan Fried Cod

Preparing time: 15 minutes

Serves: 4

Ingredients:

- 3 tbsp. of ghee
- 4 cod fillets (⅓ lb. each)
- 6 minced garlic cloves

Optional:

- Garlic powder
- Salt

Directions:

1. Melt the ghee and add half of the garlic into a skillet.
2. Arrange the fillets in the pan using medium-high heat. Sprinkle with the garlic pepper and the salt.
3. Once it turns white halfway up its side, turn it over and add the remainder of the

minced garlic. Continue cooking until it flakes easily.

4. Serve with some ghee/garlic from the pan.

Nutritional Information Per Serving (**Calories: 160 | Total Fats: 7g | Net Carbs: 1g | Protein: 21g | Fiber: 7.3g**)

82. Grilled Salmon

Preparing time: 25 minutes

Serves: 4

Ingredients:

- 1 ½ lbs. salmon fillets
- Garlic powder, to taste
- Salt, to taste
- Lemon pepper, to taste
- ⅓ cup of brown sugar
- ⅓ cup of soy sauce/amino
- ⅓ cup of water
- ¼ cup of vegetable oil

Directions:

1. Prepare the fillets with the salt, garlic powder and lemon pepper
2. Stir the brown sugar, amino, oil and water until the sugar has dissolved.

3. Toss the salmon into a Ziploc-type bag with the mixture. Put in the fridge for a minimum of 2 hours.

4. Warm up the grill to medium heat and lightly grease the surface.

5. Discard the marinade and grill the salmon for 6 to 8 minutes for each side. It should flake easily when shredded with a fork.

Nutritional Information Per Serving (Calories: 318 | Total Fats: 20.1g | Net Carbs: 13.2g | Protein: 20.5g | Fiber: 7.3g)

83. Sushi

Preparing time: 20 minutes

Serves: 4

Ingredients:

- 5 oz. smoked salmon/any seafood
- 16 oz. cauliflower
- 1 cucumber (6 inches)
- 6 oz. of softened cream cheese
- 1 tbsp. of soy sauce/coconut aminos
- 1-2 tbsp. of unseasoned rice vinegar
- 5 Nori sheets
- ½ med. avocado

Directions:

1. Pulse the cauliflower into rice-sized bits.
2. Cut up the cucumber first – end to end. Hold it upright and slice off each side. Trash the middle piece (or use it in a salad). Also, slice 2 side pieces into strips. Put in the refrigerator.
3. Prepare a hot pan and cook the cauliflower rice. Sprinkle with approximately one tablespoon of the aminos.

4. When done, add the rice to a bowl with the cream cheese and vinegar. Stir well and place in the fridge.

5. Slice ½ of the avocado into strips. Scoop the shell.

6. Place a nori sheet on a bamboo roller covered with saran wrap. Spread the mixture on the nori sheet, add the fillings and roll. Be sure it's tight.

Nutritional Information Per Serving (Calories: 353 | Total Fats: 25.7g | Net Carbs: 5.7g | Protein: 18.3g | Fiber: 7.3g)

84. Walnut Crusted Salmon

Preparing time: 20 minutes

Serves: 4

Ingredients:

- 2 tbsp. of sugar-free maple syrup
- ½ cup of walnuts
- 1 tbsp. of dijon mustard
- 2 (3 oz.) salmon fillets
- ¼ tsp. of dill
- 1 tbsp. of olive oil
- Salt and pepper, to taste

Directions:

1. Pre-heat the oven to 350°F.
2. Combine the mustard, syrup and nuts in the processor and pulse until it has a consistency of paste.
3. Pour the oil into a skillet and let sit until it gets hot. Sear about 3 minutes.

Spread the walnut mixture on the top side of the fillets.

4. Move them to the oven and bake for approximately 7 to 8 minutes.

Nutritional Information Per Serving **(Calories: 373 | Total Fats: 43g | Net Carbs: 3g | Protein: 20g | Fiber: 7.3g)**

85. One-Pot Shrimp Alfredo

Preparing time: 35 minutes

Serves: 4

Ingredients:

- 1 lb. raw shrimp
- 1 tbsp. of salted butter
- 4 oz. of cubed cream cheese
- ½ cup of whole milk
- 1 tsp. of salt
- 1 tsp. of dried basil
- 1 tbsp. of garlic powder
- ½ cup of shredded parmesan cheese
- ¼ cup of baby kale
- 5 whole sun-dried tomatoes – in strips

Directions:

1. Heat up the butter (medium heat) in a pan. Toss in the shrimp and lower the heat to medium-low. After 30 seconds, flip the shrimp and cook until slightly pink. Blend in the cream cheese.

2. Increase the heat and pour in the milk, stirring frequently.

3. Sprinkle with the salt, basil and garlic. Empty the parmesan cheese in and mix well. Simmer until the sauce has thickened. Lastly, fold in the kale/spinach and dried tomatoes.

4. Serve steaming hot.

Nutritional Information Per Serving (Calories: 297.83 | Total Fats: 17.55g | Net Carbs: 6.51g | Protein: 22.93g | Fiber: 7.3g)

86. Loaded Tuna Fish Salad

Preparing time: 15 minutes

Serves: 4

Ingredients:

- 1 small can tuna
- 1 large chopped boiled egg
- 2 bacon slices
- 1 tbsp. of mayonnaise
- 1 tbsp. of chopped onion
- 1 tbsp. of sour cream
- 2 tsp. of dijon mustard
- ¼ tsp. of dill

Directions:

1. Chop the onion, cook the bacon and boil the egg.
2. Drain the tuna and add it to a container. Toss in the egg and onion.
3. Blend in the rest of the fixings. Top with the crumbled bacon and enjoy!

Nutritional Information Per Serving **(Calories: 298 | Total Fats: 23g | Net Carbs: 1g | Protein: 21g | Fiber: 7.3g)**

87. Tuna Tartare

Preparing time: 15 minutes

Serves: 4

Ingredients:

- 1 avocado
- 1 lb. tuna steak
- 3 scallion stalks
- 1 jalapeno
- 2 tbsp. of sesame seed oil
- 2 tbsp. of olive oil
- 1 tbsp. of soy sauce
- 1 tbsp. of sriracha
- 1 tbsp. of mayonnaise
- ½ lime
- 1 tsp. of sesame seeds
- 2 Persian cucumbers

Directions:

1. Dice the avocado and steak into ¼-inch pieces.
2. Dice the jalapeno and scallion finely into another dish. Empty juice of the lime

and mix with the remainder of the ingredients.

3. Slice the cucumber, add the mixture on top and serve with a drizzle of seeds. Enjoy!

Nutritional Information Per Serving (Calories: 287 | Total Fats: 24.5g | Net Carbs: 4g | Protein: 56.5g | Fiber: 7.3g

88. Chipotle Fish Tacos

Preparing time: 35 minutes

Serves: 4

Ingredients:

- ½ small yellow onion, diced
- 2 pressed cloves of garlic
- 1 fresh jalapeno, chopped
- 2 tbsp. of olive oil
- 4 oz. chipotle peppers in adobo sauce
- 2 tbsp. of mayonnaise
- 2 tbsp. of butter
- 4 low-carb tortillas
- 1 lb. haddock fillets

Directions:

1. Reduce the temperature to medium. Toss in the garlic and jalapeno. Stir another 2 minutes.
2. Chop and add the chipotles, along with the adobo sauce into the pan.
3. Drop the butter, mayonnaise and fish into the pan and cook about 8 minutes.

4. Make the Tacos: Fry the tortilla for approximately 2 minutes for each side. Chill and shape them with the fix mixture.

Nutritional Information Per Serving **(Calories: 300 | Total Fats: 20g | Net Carbs: 7g | Protein: 24g | Fiber: 7.3g)**

89. Bell Pepper Basil Pizza

Preparing time: 45 minutes

Serves: 2

Ingredients:

Pizza Base:

- 6 oz. mozzarella cheese
- 2 tbsp. of fresh parmesan cheese
- 2 tbsp. of cream cheese
- 2 tbsp. of Psyllium husk
- 1 tsp. of Italian seasoning
- 1 large egg
- ½ tsp. of black pepper
- ½ tsp. of salt

Toppings:

- 4 oz. shredded cheddar cheese
- ¼ cup of marinara sauce
- 1 med. vine ripened tomato
- 2-3 med. bell peppers
- 2-3 tbsp. of fresh basil, chopped

Directions:

1. Pre-heat the oven to 400°F.

2. Melt the cheese in the microwave until melted and pliable or for 40-50 seconds.

3. Add the remainder of the pizza base fixings to the cheese – mixing well with your hands. Flatten the dough to form the two circular pizzas.

4. Bake 10 minutes. Remove and add the toppings. Take for about 8-10 additional minutes.

5. Let it cool and serve.

Nutritional Information Per Serving (Calories: 211.5 | Total Fats: 31.32g (per ½ of a pizza per serving) | Net Carbs: 6.46g | Protein: 22.26g | Fiber: 7.3g)

90. Cheesy Brussels Sprouts

Preparing time: 40 minutes

Serves: 4

Ingredients:

- 16 oz. of brussels sprout
- 5 bacon slices
- 6 oz. of cheddar cheese

Directions:

1. Prepare the bacon and set aside on towels to drain (reserve the grease).
2. Rinse the sprouts and shred with a food processor.
3. Fry the sprouts in the grease until crispy.

Nutritional Information Per Serving **(Calories: 256 | Total Fats: 20g | Net Carbs: 2g | Protein: 16g | Fiber: 7.3g)**

Chapter 11: Desserts

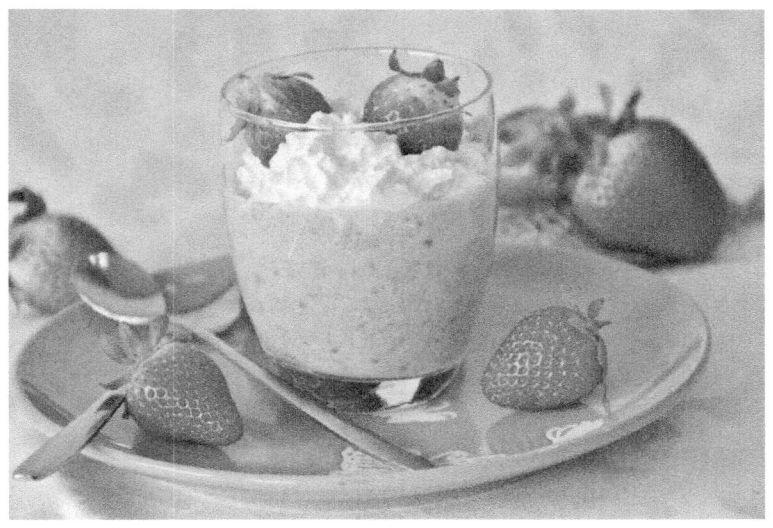

90. Cheesy Brussels Sprouts

Preparing time: 40 minutes

Serves: 4

Ingredients:

- 16 oz. of brussels sprout
- 5 bacon slices
- 6 oz. of cheddar cheese

Directions:

4. Prepare the bacon and set aside on towels to drain (reserve the grease).
5. Rinse the sprouts and shred with a food processor.
6. Fry the sprouts in the grease until crispy.

Nutritional Information Per Serving **(Calories: 256 | Total Fats: 20g | Net Carbs: 2g | Protein: 16g | Fiber: 7.3g)**

91. Mini Chocolate Cakes

Preparing time: 35 minutes

Serves: 2

Ingredients:

- 2 tbsp. of heavy cream
- ¼ cup of baking cocoa
- ½ tsp. of baking powder
- 2 tbsp. of Splenda
- 1 tsp. of vanilla
- 2 eggs

Directions:

1. Stir everything together in a bowl. Grease two ramekins and split the batter between the two.
2. Place a cup of water to the pot and set in the trivet.
3. Set the ramekins and lock the lid in place the set the cooker on high for 9 minutes.
4. Quick release the pressure and then flip the cakes onto a plate.

Nutritional Information Per Serving (Calories: 120 | Total Fats: 4.8g | Net Carbs: 7g | Protein: 0.8g | Fiber: 7.3g

92. Poached Eggs

Preparing time: 5 minutes

Serves: 4

Ingredients:

- 1 cup of water
- 4-5 eggs

Directions:

1. Set your trivet into the pot and add a cup of water.
2. Coat silicone cups with nonstick spray and crack an egg into each.
3. Set the cups into your pot.
4. Quick release the pressure and take off the lid. Lift out the cups and enjoy.

Nutritional Information Per Serving (**Calories: 70 | Total Fats: 5g | Net Carbs: 0.4g | Protein: 6.3g | Fiber: 7.3g**

93. Ricotta Lemon Cheesecake

Preparing time: 25 minutes

Serves: 6

Ingredients:

- 2 eggs
- ½ tsp. of lemon extract
- 1 lemon, juice and zest
- ⅓ cup of ricotta
- ¼ cup of trivia
- 8 oz. of cream cheese

Topping:

- 1 tsp. of Truvia
- 2 tbsp. of sour cream

Directions:

1. Beat all the ingredients together except for the eggs until there are no lumps. Mix the eggs. Don't overbeat. Pour this into a greased springform pan and place foil over the top.

2. Add two cups of water and the trivet in your pot and set on the cake. Lock the lid and set on high for 30 minutes. Let pressure release naturally.

3. Stir together the Truvia and sour cream. Spread this over the warm cake and refrigerate for 6 to 8 hours.

Nutritional Information Per Serving (Calories: 190 | Total Fats: 9g | Net Carbs: 6g | Protein: 8g | Fiber: 7.3g)

94. Wheat Belly Yogurt

Preparing time: 20 minutes

Serves: 4

Ingredients:

- 2 tbsp. of full-fat yogurt with live cultures
- 16 oz. of heavy whipping cream

Directions:

1. Stir the ingredients together in a glass bowl.
2. Place in your Instant Pot and follow the yogurt making directions.

Nutritional Information Per Serving (Calories: 149 | Total Fats: 8g | Net Carbs: 7g | Protein: 8.5g | Fiber: 7.3g)

95. Eggs in a Cup

Preparing time: 5 minutes

Serves: 4

Ingredients:

- Pepper and salt, to taste
- ¼ cup of half & half
- 2 tbsp. of cilantro
- ½ cup of cheddar cheese
- ½ cup of shredded cheddar cheese
- 1 cup of diced veggies
- 4 eggs

Directions:

1. Combine the coriander, pepper, salt, half & half, cheese, vegetables and eggs and divide into 4-pint jars. Loosely place on lids.

2. Add 2 cups water to the pot and trivet. Set the jars. Lock the lid and set the

cooker on high for 5 minutes. Once done, release the pressure.

3. Add shredded cheddar cheese and broil for a few minutes.

Nutritional Information Per Serving **(Calories: 115 | Total Fats: 9g | Net Carbs: 2g | Protein: 9g | Fiber: 7.3g)**

96. Vanilla Bean Cheesecake

Preparing time: 10 minutes

Serves: 8

Ingredients:

- Raspberry jam
- 1 vanilla bean, scraped
- ½ cup of swerve
- 1 tsp. of vanilla
- 1 eggs
- 16 oz. of cultured cream cheese

Directions:

1. Whisk everything together in a blender. Add to a spring form pan and cover with foil. Add 2 cups of water to the pot and set on a rack.

2. Ease in the pan and lock the lid then set the cooker on high for 20 minutes. Once done, naturally release pressure.

3. Take out of the pot and let it cool to room temperature. Refrigerate at least an hour before serving.

Nutritional Information Per Serving (Calories: 100 | Total Fats: 10g | Net Carbs: 8g | Protein: 6g | Fiber: 7.3g)

97. Greek Yogurt

Preparing time: 20 minutes

Serves: 14

Ingredients:

- 2 tbsp. yogurt starter
- 1 gallon of milk

Directions:

1. Place juice in the cooker. Cover the lid and press the yogurt button and adjust to boil. Whisk now and then during the cooking time.

2. Check the temperature once done, should be 180°F. If not, cook again. Once hot, take the pot out and set in cold water and whisk until it cools to 95°F-110°F.

3. Remove a bit of milk and mix the starter. Mix back in. Place back in the Instant Pot and place the lid and press yogurt, adjust to 8:00.

4. Remove the pot and refrigerate until cold. Don't stir.

5. Strain milk through yogurt strainer for the Greek yogurt

Nutritional Information Per Serving (Calories: 220 | Total Fats: 11g | Net Carbs: 9g | Protein: 20g | Fiber: 7.3g

98. Garlic Spread

Preparing time: 10 minutes

Serves: Varies

Ingredients:

- Salt
- 2 tbsp. of olive oil
- 5-6 garlic heads

Directions:

1. Place ⅔ cup water in your pot and set in a steamer basket. Cut the top off the garlic head.
2. Set the garlic heads and drizzle with oil. Lock the lid, then set the cooker to high pressure for 10 minutes.
3. Reduce the pressure and remove the garlic then sprinkle with salt.
4. Once cool, remove cloves and mash together with a fork. Keep in the fridge.

Nutrition Information Per Serving **(Calories: 34 | Total Fats: 2g | Net Carbs: 5g | Protein: 0g | Fiber: 7.3g)**

99. Peanut Butter Cheesecake

Preparing time: 15 minutes

Serves: 8

Ingredients:

- 1 tsp. of vanilla
- 1 tbsp. of cocoa
- ½ cup of swerve
- 2 tbsp. of powdered peanut butter
- 2 eggs
- 16 oz. of cream cheese

Directions:

1. Blend eggs and cream cheese, and then add all the other ingredients. Place in 4 oz. or 8 oz. jars and loosely place the lid.
2. Place a cup of water to the pot and set the trivet. Set the jars, lock the lid and set the cooker on high for 15-18 minutes.
3. Once done, release pressure and remove.

Nutritional Information Per Serving (Calories: 191 | Total Fats: 16g | Net Carbs: 5g | Protein: 6g | Fiber: 7.3g)

100. Pumpkin Pecan Cake

Preparing time: 20 minutes

Serves: 10

Ingredients:

- ¼ tsp. of salt
- 1 tsp. of ginger
- ¼ cup of protein powder
- 4 eggs
- 1 cup of pumpkin puree
- ¼ tsp. of cloves
- 1 tsp. of vanilla
- 1 ½ tsp. of cinnamon
- ¼ cup of butter, melted
- 2 tsp. of baking powder
- ⅓ cup of coconut flour
- ¾ cup of swerve
- 1 ½ cups of raw pecans

Directions:

1. Grease your pot, then grind pecans in a processor. Place in a bowl and mix the spices, sweetener and coconut.

2. Mix the vanilla, butter, eggs and pumpkin.

3. Spread into the pot. Place the lid and set to slow cook for 2 ½ hours. Enjoy.

Nutritional Information Per Serving (Calories: 250 | Total Fats: 17g | Net Carbs: 8g | Protein: 7g | Fiber: 7.3g)

101. Chocolate Cream

Preparing time: 10 minutes

Serves: 4

Ingredients:

- 2 cups heavy cream
- ¼ cup of unsweetened dark chocolate, chopped
- 3 eggs
- 1 tsp. of orange zest
- 1 tsp. of stevia powder
- 1 tsp. of vanilla extract
- ½ tsp. of salt

Directions:

1. Plug in your instant pot and press the 'Sauté' button. Add heavy cream, chopped chocolate, stevia powder, vanilla extract, orange zest and salt. Stir well and simmer until the chocolate has completely melted.

2. Press the 'Cancel' button and crack eggs, one at the time, stirring constantly. Remove from the instant pot.

3. Transfer the mixture to 4 mason jars with loose lids.

4. Pour 2 cups of water in your instant pot and set the trivet in the stainless-steel insert. Add jars and seal the lid.

5. Set the steam release handle and press the 'Manual' button. Set the timer for 10 minutes.

6. When done, perform a quick release by moving the steam valve to the 'Venting' position.

7. Open the lid and remove the jars. Chill to room temperature and then transfer to the refrigerator.

8. Top with some whipped cream before serving.

Nutritional Information Per Serving **(Calories: 267 | Total Fats: 26.2g | Net Carbs: 2.4g | Protein 5.6g | Fiber: 0.2g)**

102. Butter Pancakes

Preparing time: 10 minutes

Serves: 6

Ingredients:

- 2 cups of cream cheese
- 2 cups of almond flour
- 6 large eggs
- ¼ tsp. of salt
- 2 tbsp. of butter
- ¼ tsp. of ground ginger
- ½ tsp. of cinnamon powder

Directions:

1. Mix cream cheese, butter and eggs
2. Slowly add flour beating continually.
3. Finally, add salt, ginger and cinnamon. Continue to beat until fully incorporated.
4. Plug in your instant pot and press the 'Sauté' button. Grease the stainless-

steel insert with the remaining butter and heat up.

5. Pour in about ½ cup of the batter and cook for 2-3 minutes or until golden color. Repeat the process with the remaining dough.

6. Serve warm.

Nutritional Information Per Serving (Calories: 132 | Total Fats: 40.2g | Net Carbs: 3.5g | Protein: 14.2g |Fiber: 1g)

103. Raspberry Cookies

Preparing time: 15 minutes

Serves: 6

Ingredients:

- 1 ½ cups of almond flour
- ¾ tsp. of baking powder
- ¼ tsp. of baking soda
- ¼ cup of unsweetened almond milk
- 2 large eggs
- ¼ cup of almond butter
- ¼ cup of swerve
- 1 tbsp. of raw almonds, chopped
- 1 tsp. of raspberry extract

Directions:

1. Beat eggs and raspberry extract and swerve gently pour in the milk and almond butter. Continue to beat for 1 minute.

2. Finally, add the remaining ingredients and mix until thoroughly combined.

3. Line some parchment paper over a small baking dish and plug in your instant pot. Pour in 1 cup of water and

set the trivet at the bottom of the steel insert.

4. Spoon 1 tbsp. of the mixture onto the prepared baking pan and flatten the surface with your hands.

5. Loosely cover with some aluminum foil and seal the lid. Set the steam release handle to the 'Sealing' position and press the 'Manual' button. Set the timer for 15 minutes.

6. When you hear the cooker's end signal, perform a quick release and open the lid.

7. Remove the pan and transfer cookies to a wire rack to cool completely before serving.

Nutritional Information Per Serving **(Calories: 78 | Total Fats: 6g | Net Carbs: 1.4g | Protein 4g | Fiber: 1g)**

104. Vanilla Mousse with Chocolate Sauce

Preparing time: 20 minutes

Serves: 4

Ingredients:

- 2 cups of cream cheese
- 1 cup of whipped cream
- 4 tbsp. of coconut oil
- 1 tsp. of vanilla extract
- ¼ cup of swerve
- 4 tbsp. of unsweetened cocoa powder
- ¼ cup of unsweetened dark chocolate
- ¼ cup of unsweetened almond milk

Directions:

1. In a container, combine cream cheese, whipped cream, 2 tbsp. of coconut oil, cocoa powder, vanilla extract and swerve. With a paddle attachment on, beat well on high speed until light and fluffy mixture. Divide between 4 serving cups and refrigerate.

2. Meanwhile, plug in your instant pot and press the 'Sauté' button. Grease the stainless-steel insert with the remaining

coconut oil and heat up. Add chocolate and gently melt, stirring constantly. Pour in the milk and simmer for 5 minutes.

3. Press the cancel button and remove the chocolate sauce. Drizzle the chilled mousse with the sauce and serve immediately.

Nutritional Information Per Serving **(Calories: 253 | Total Fats: 66.3g | Net Carbs: 5.2g | Protein 10.2g | Fiber: 0.8g)**

105. Sweet Almond Buns

Preparing time: 20 minutes

Serves: 6

Ingredients:

- 1 cup of almond flour
- ½ cup of coconut flour
- ⅓ cup psyllium husk powder
- ½ cup of cocoa powder, unsweetened
- 1 tsp. baking soda
- 4 large eggs
- 1 tbsp. of raw almonds, finely chopped
- ½ cup of swerve
- ½ cup of almond butter

Directions:

1. Mix all the dry ingredients and add eggs, one at the time, and beat well with a dough hook attachment. Now add almond butter and continue to beat until smooth dough.

2. Transfer the dough to a lightly floured surface and divide into six equal balls. Press each ball with your hands until about 1-inch thick. Set aside.

3. Line some parchment paper over a small baking pan and plug in your instant pot. Pour in 1 cup of water and place the trivet at the bottom.

4. Gently place the buns in your baking pan and loosely cover with aluminum foil. Place the pan in the pot and seal the lid. Set the steam release handle to the 'Sealing' position and press the 'Manual' button.

5. Set the timer for 30 minutes.

6. When done, release the pressure naturally for 15 minutes and then move the pressure valve to the 'Venting' position to release any remaining tension.

7. Open the lid and remove the pan. Cool to room temperature and transfer buns to a wire rack to cool completely.

Nutritional Information Per Serving (Calories: 130 | Total Fats: 8.2g | Net Carbs: 4.2g | Protein: 7.7g | Fiber: 6.1g)

106. Cocoa Patties

Preparing time: 25 minutes

Serves: 4

Ingredients:

- 1 cup of cream cheese
- 4 large eggs
- 2 tbsp. of swerve
- ¼ cup of cocoa powder, unsweetened
- 2 tbsp. of coconut oil plus, for frying
- 1 tsp. of vanilla extract

Directions:

1. Mix all the ingredients. With a paddle attachment on, beat well on high speed until thoroughly combined.
2. Plug in your instant pot and press the 'Sauté' button. Grease the stainless-steel insert with some oil and heat up.
3. Pour in about ¼ cup of the cocoa butter and cook for 3-4 minutes, or until golden-brown color.
4. Optionally, top with some whipped cream.

Nutritional Information Per Serving (Calories: 156 | Total Fats: 45.6g | Net Carbs: 2.1g | Protein: 10.7g | Fiber: 0g)

107. Easy Almond Bars

Preparing time: 20 minutes

Serves: 3

Ingredients:

- ¼ cup of almond flour
- ¼ cup of coconut flour
- ½ cup of coconut oil
- 2 tbsp. of almond butter
- ¼ tsp. of salt
- 3 tbsp. of swerve
- 1 tsp. of vanilla extract
- 2 large eggs

Directions:

1. Plug in your instant pot and set the trivet. Pour in 1 cup of water at the bottom of the stainless-steel insert and set aside.
2. Combine the ingredients in a food processor and process until 'sandy' texture.
3. Line a small baking pan with some parchment paper and add the dough. Press well with the palm of your hands and gently place in your instant pot.

4. Cover with some parchment paper and seal the lid. Set the steam release handle to the 'Sealing' position and press the 'Manual' button.

5. Set the timer for 15 minutes.

6. When done, release the pressure naturally and open the lid. Using oven mitts carefully remove the pan from your instant pot and chill to room temperature.

7. Slice into 6 bars and refrigerate for at least an hour before serving.

Nutritional Information Per Serving (Calories: 253 | Total Fats: 25.7g | Net Carbs: 1.5g | Protein: 4.6g | Fiber: 1.4g)

108. Pumpkin Pie Pancakes

Preparing time: 25 minutes

Serves: 4

Ingredients:

- 1 cup of pumpkin puree
- 3 large eggs
- 2 tbsp. of swerve
- ¾ cup of almond flour
- 4 tbsp. of almond milk, unsweetened
- 1 tsp. of pumpkin pie seasoning
- ¼ tsp. of salt
- 2 tsp. of baking powder

Directions:

1. In a large mixing bowl, combine eggs, swerve, pumpkin pie seasoning and almond milk.
2. With a whisking attachment on, beat well on high speed. Gradually add flour, salt, baking powder and pumpkin pie seasoning.
3. Continue to mix for another 2 minutes.
4. Finally, add the pumpkin puree and mix well again.

5. Plug in your instant pot and press the 'Sauté' button. Grease the stainless-steel insert with some oil and heat up. Add about ¼ cup of the batter and cook for 3 minutes.

Nutritional Information Per Serving (Calories: 143 | Total Fats: 10g | Net Carbs: 5.7g | Protein: 6.9g | Fiber: 2.7

109. Coconut Brownies with Raspberries

Preparing time: 30 minutes

Serves: 6

Ingredients:

- 1 ½ cup of almond flour
- ½ cup of fresh raspberries
- ½ cup of shredded coconut
- ¼ cup of swerve
- 1 tsp. of baking soda
- ½ cup of coconut oil
- 2 large eggs

Directions:

1. Combine almond flour, shredded coconut, baking soda and swerve. Mix well and add coconut oil and eggs. With a dough hook attachment, beat well until thoroughly combined. Fold in raspberries and set aside.

2. Line a small baking pan with some parchment paper and add the mixture. Press well with your hands and tightly wrap with aluminum foil.

3. Plug in your instant pot and pour in 1 cup of water. Set the trivet and place the baking pan on top.

4. Seal the lid and set the steam release handle. Press the 'Manual' button and set the timer for 20 minutes.

5. When you hear the cooker's end signal, perform a quick release and open the lid.

6. Remove the baking pan and cool completely before slicing.

7. Optionally, sprinkle with some more shredded coconut.

Nutritional Information Per Serving **(Calories: 251 | Total Fats: 25.5g | Net Carbs: 1.9g | Protein: 4g | Fiber: 2g)**

110. Chocolate Chip Cookies

Preparing time: 30 minutes

Serves: 10

Ingredients:

- ½ cup of almond flour
- ¼ cup of flax meal
- ¼ cup of coconut flour
- ½ cup of almond butter
- ¼ cup of coconut oil
- ¼ tsp. of salt
- ¼ cup of swerve
- 3 large eggs
- 1 tsp. of vanilla extract
- ¼ cup of dark chocolate chips, unsweetened

Directions:

1. Mix all the dry ingredients and transfer to a food processor along with almond butter, coconut oil, eggs and vanilla extract. Process until sandy texture.
2. Transfer the mixture to a lightly floured work surface and fold in chocolate

chips. Knead with your hands and shape 10 balls.

3. Line a baking pan with some parchment paper and place cookies. Plug in your instant pot and pour in 1 cup of water. Set the trivet and place the pan on top.

4. Seal the lid and set the steam release handle to the 'Sealing' position. Press the 'Manual' button and set the timer for 15 minutes.

5. When done, release the pressure naturally and open the lid.

6. Transfer cookies to a wire rack and cool completely before serving.

Nutritional Information Per Serving **(Calories: 133 | Total Fats: 11.2g | Net Carbs: 3.2g | Protein: 4.2g | Fiber: 3g)**

111. Vanilla Cream

Preparing time: 10 minutes

Serves: 4

Ingredients:

- 8 large eggs
- ¾ cup of unsweetened almond milk
- 1 ½ cups of heavy cream
- 1 tsp. of vanilla extract
- 1 vanilla bean
- 4 tbsp. of swerve

Directions:

1. Cut the vanilla bean lengthwise and scrape out the seeds. Place in a mixing bowl along with the remaining ingredients.

2. With a whisking attachment on, beat the mixture for 2 minutes on high speed and transfer into four ramekins. Tightly wrap with aluminum foil and set aside.

3. Plug in your instant pot and pour in 2 cups of water. Set the trivet at the bottom of the stainless-steel insert and carefully place the ramekins on top.

4. Seal the lid and set the steam release handle to the 'Sealing' position. Press the 'Manual' button and set the timer for 15 minutes.

5. When done, perform a quick release by moving the pressure valve to the 'Venting' position.

6. Open the lid and carefully remove the ramekins from your instant pot.

7. Cool to room temperature without removing the aluminum foil.

8. Transfer to the fridge and cool completely before serving.

Nutritional Information Per Serving (Calories: 209 | Total Fats: 27.3g | Net Carbs: 2.3g | Protein: 13.7g | Fiber: 0.2g)

112. Cheesecake with Warm Chocolate Sauce

Preparing time: 20 minutes

Serves: 10

Ingredients:

- 1 ½ cups of almond flour
- ⅓ cup of shredded coconut
- ⅓ cup of coconut oil
- 3 large eggs
- 2 tbsp. of raw almonds, minced
- 3 cups of cream cheese
- 1 cup of whipped cream
- ¼ cup of plain Greek yogurt
- 1 tsp. vanilla extract
- ¼ cup of swerve
- ½ cup of dark chocolate, unsweetened
- ¼ cup of almond milk, unsweetened

Directions:

1. First, prepare the crust. Combine almond flour, coconut flour, salt, and minced almonds in a large bowl. Mix well and add coconut oil and eggs. With

a paddle attachment on, beat well on medium speed until fully incorporated.

2. Brush a 7-inches baking pan with some coconut oil and line with parchment paper. Add the batter and flatten the surface with a kitchen spatula. Loosely cover with aluminum foil.

3. Plug in your instant pot and pour in 1 cup of water. Set the trivet and place the pan on top. Seal the lid and set the steam release handle to the 'Sealing' position. Press the 'Manual' button and set the timer for 15 minutes.

4. When done, release the pressure naturally for 15 minutes and open the lid. Carefully remove the pan and chill for a while.

5. Meanwhile, prepare the cream layer. Combine cream cheese, whipped cream, Greek yogurt, vanilla extract and swerve in a large mixing bowl.

Nutritional Information Per Serving
(Calories: 129 | Total Fats: 2.3g | Net Carbs: 2.2g | Protein 10.7g | Fiber: 1.2g)

113. Peanut Butter Brownies

Preparing time: 20 minutes

Serves: 8

Ingredients:

- 1 cup of almond flour
- 1 cup of flax meal
- 1 cup of peanut butter
- 1 cup of unsweetened dark chocolate
- 2 tsp. of baking powder
- 2 eggs
- ¼ tsp. of salt

Directions:

1. Line a small baking pan with some parchment paper and set aside.
2. Combine the ingredients in a food processor and process until smooth. Transfer the mixture to the prepared baking pan and tightly cover with aluminum foil.
3. Plug in the instant pot and pour in 1 cup of water. Set the trivet at the bottom of the stainless-steel insert and set aside. Place the pan on top and seal the lid.

4. Set the steam release handle and press the 'Manual' button. Set the timer for 25 minutes.

5. When done, perform a quick release and open the lid. Remove the pan carefully and chill to room temperature before slicing.

Nutritional Information Per Serving (Calories: 210 | Total Fats: 34g | Net Carbs: 6.7g | Protein: 17.4g | Fiber: 11.6g)

114. Chocolate Chip Keto Brownies

Preparing time: 20 minutes

Serves: 8

Ingredients:

- 1 ½ cups of almond flour
- ¼ cup of coconut flakes, unsweetened
- 2 tbsp. of chia seeds
- 3 large eggs
- ½ cup of coconut oil, melted
- ¼ cup of swerve
- ¼ cup of unsweetened dark chocolate chips

Directions:

1. Line an 8x8 inches pan with some parchment paper.
2. Mix well and add eggs, one at the time, mixing continuously. Finally, add coconut oil and chocolate chips.
3. Transfer to the prepared baking pan and flatten the surface with your hands. Loosely cover with some aluminum foil and set aside.
4. Plug in your instant pot set the trivet at the bottom of the stainless-steel insert.

Pour in 1 cup of water and place the pan on top.

5. Seal the lid and set the steam release handle to the 'Sealing' position. Press the 'Manual' button and set the timer for 20 minutes.

6. When done, perform a quick pressure release and open the lid. Carefully remove the pan and chill to room temperature.

7. Cut into 8 brownies and cool completely before serving.

Nutritional Information Per Serving **(Calories: 237 | Total Fats: 23.1g | Net Carbs: 1.9g | Protein: 5.1g | Fiber: 2.8g)**

115. Raspberry Yogurt with Avocado

Preparing time: 10 minutes

Serves: 5

Ingredients:

- 2 cups of whipping cream, sugar-free
- 1 cup of plain yogurt
- 1 tbsp. of powdered stevia
- 1 cup of fresh raspberries
- 1 tbsp. of vanilla extract, sugar-free
- 1 tbsp. of arrowroot powder
- ¼ cup of avocado, cut into chunks
- 1 oz. pack of cherry gelatin

Directions:

1. Combine raspberries, stevia, vanilla extract, and arrowroot powder in the stainless-steel insert of your instant pot. Lock the lid and adjust the steam release handle. Press "Manual" button and set the timer for 15 minutes. Cook on high pressure.

2. In a large mixing bowl, whisk together whipping cream and yogurt. Beat for 2 minutes on high speed and set aside.

3. Open the pot and transfer the mixture to a bowl with cream. Using a hand mixer beat well for one more minute. Chill completely.

4. Peel the avocado and remove the pit. Cut into chunks and set aside.

5. Add gelatin to your instant pot and pour in 1 cup of water. Press the 'Sauté' button and gently bring it to a boil, stirring constantly. Cook for 2-3 minutes, or until gelatin dissolves completely.

6. Divide the raspberry yogurt between 5 glasses and top each with avocado chunks. Top each with gelatin and freeze for 20 minutes before serving.

Nutritional Information Per Serving **(Calories: 218 | Total Fats: 17g | Net Carbs: 8.6g | Protein: 4.3g | Fiber: 2.1g)**

116. Cherry Pudding

Preparing time: 15 minutes

Serves: 5

Ingredients:

- ¾ cup of whipped cream
- ¾ cup of almond milk, unsweetened
- 4 egg whites
- 3 tsp. of powdered stevia
- 1 tsp. of cherry extract, sugar-free
- ¼ tsp. of xanthan gum

Directions:

1. Combine almond milk, cream and egg whites. Beat well on high, for 3 minutes. Pour the mixture into five ramekins.

2. Plug in your instant pot and pour 2 cups of water into the stainless-steel insert. Position a trivet at the bottom and place the ramekins on top. Securely lock the lid and adjust the steam release handle. Press "Manual" button and set the timer for 3 minutes. Cook on high pressure.

3. When you hear the cooker's end signal, press "Cancel" button and release the pressure naturally.

4. Open the pot and chill the pudding to room temperature. Refrigerate for 1 hour before serving.

Nutritional Information Per Serving (Calories: 153 | Total Fats: 14.2g | Net Carbs: 2g | Protein: 4.5g | Fiber: 5.8g)

117. Creamy Raspberry Cake

Preparing time: 10 minutes

Serves: 8

Ingredients:

- ½ cup of coconut flour
- ¼ cup of heavy cream
- ½ cup of fresh raspberries
- 5 egg yolks
- ¼ cup of butter
- 3 tsp. of powdered stevia
- 1 tsp. of baking powder
- 1 tsp. of vanilla extract, sugar-free
- ¼ cup of coconut oil

Directions:

1. Combine all dry ingredients except raspberries in a large mixing bowl and mix until combined. Add all wet ingredients and beat until thoroughly combined.

2. Line a 6-inch spring form pan with some parchment paper and pour in the batter. Spread the raspberries on top by tucking them into the mixture.

3. Plug in your instant pot and pour in 2 cups of water. Position a trivet in the stainless-steel insert and place the pan on top.

4. Securely close the lid and adjust the steam release handle. Press the "Manual" button and set the timer for 10 minutes. Cook on high pressure.

5. When done, press "Cancel" button and perform a quick release of the pressure by turning the valve to the venting position.

6. Open the pot and let it chill for a while before serving.

Nutritional Information Per Serving **(Calories: 222 | Total Fats: 18.3g | Net Carbs: 5.3g | Protein: 3.9g | Fiber: 6.5g)**

118. Strawberry Chocolate Fudge

Preparing time: 25 minutes

Serves: 8

Ingredients:

- 2 cups of almond flour
- ½ cup of dark chocolate, unsweetened
- ½ cup of raw cocoa powder
- 2 tsp. of powdered stevia
- ½ cup of almond milk, unsweetened
- 1 tsp. of baking powder
- 1 tsp. of baking soda
- 5 eggs
- 1 tsp. of strawberry extract, sugar-free
- ½ tsp. of salt

Directions:

1. Mix all dry ingredients until combined. Now, add all the remaining ingredients. With a paddle attachment on, beat until all well incorporated.

2. Plug in your instant pot and pour in 2 cups of water. Position a trivet in the stainless-steel insert. Pour in the previously prepared mixture into a

greased spring form pan. Place the pan on top of a trivet and close the lid.

3. Adjust the steam release handle and set the timer for 15 minutes. Cook on high pressure.

4. Once done, press "Cancel" button and turn off the pot. Open the lid and let it chill for a while before serving.

Nutritional information Per Serving (Calories: 242 | Total Fats: 18.6g | Net Carbs: 6.2g | Protein: 8.5g | Fiber: 4.9g)

119. Apple Lemon Pie

Preparing time: 30 minutes

Serves: 10

Ingredients:

- 2 small Granny Smith apples, peeled and thinly sliced
- 1 cup of coconut flour
- ½ cup of almond flour
- 1 tsp. of baking powder
- ½ tsp. of salt
- 1 tbsp. of lemon juice, freshly squeezed
- 1 tsp. of lemon extract, sugar-free
- 1 tbsp. of instant gelatin
- 3 tbsp. of coconut oil, melted

Directions:

1. Combine apples, lemon extract and lemon juice in a large bowl. Mix until apple slices are well coated. Transfer all to a spring form pan lined with some parchment paper. Set aside.
2. Now, combine all dry ingredients in a large bowl and mix until combined. Add

all wet ingredients and mix with a kitchen spatula until dough is formed.

3. Plug in your instant pot and pour in 2 cups of water. Position a trivet in the stainless-steel insert. Place the pan on top and securely lock the lid. Adjust the steam release handle and set the timer for 20 minutes. Cook on high pressure.

4. Open the pot and let it chill for a while. Once cooled, turn the pan upside down and remove the parchment paper. Cut into slices and serve immediately.

Nutritional Information Per Serving **(Calories: 132 | Total Fats: 6.9g | Net Carbs: 7g | Protein: 3.2g | Fiber: 7.3g)**

120. Almond Strawberry Squares

Preparing time: 18 minutes

Serves: 8

Ingredients:

- 1 ½ cup of almond flour
- ¼ cup of almonds, ground
- 1 tbsp. of cocoa powder, unsweetened
- 1 tsp. of baking powder
- ½ cup of heavy cream
- ½ cup of almond milk
- 1 large egg
- 1 tsp. of vanilla extract

Strawberry layer:

- ½ cup of fresh strawberries, chopped
- 1 cup of whipped cream and 2 tbsp. of Greek yogurt

Directions:

1. Mix all the dry ingredients until well combined
2. In a separate bowl, whisk eggs, heavy cream and vanilla extract. Now,

combine dry and wet ingredients and mix until well incorporated.

3. Plug in your instant pot and pour in 2 cups of water. Position a trivet in the stainless-steel insert. Line a 6-inch spring form pan with some parchment paper. Spread the previously prepared mixture evenly and place the pan on top of a trivet. Securely lock the lid and adjust the steam release handle. Press the "Manual" button and set the timer for 8 minutes. Cook on high pressure.

4. When done, perform a quick release and open the pot. Carefully transfer the pan to a wire rack and let it cool completely.

5. Meanwhile, combine all strawberry layer ingredients in a food processor. Pulse until creamy. Spoon this mixture onto chilled crust. Using a kitchen spatula, spread the batter evenly. Refrigerate for 45 minutes or freeze for 20 minutes. Cut into squares before serving.

Nutritional Information Per Serving (Calories: 171 | Total Fats: 15.8g | Net Carbs: 3.2g | Protein: 3.9g |Fiber: 1.7g)

Chapter 12: 4 Weeks of Ketogenic Meal Planning

Week 1: Shopping List

- 3 avocados
- 1 can of tuna
- 10 eggs
- 1 cup of spinach
- 5 beef tenderloin steaks
- 12 oz. of cream cheese
- 10 lbs. of chicken breasts
- 1 lb. of trimmed asparagus
- Unsweetened shredded coconut
- ½ tsp. of coriander
- 2 tsp. of curry powder
- 1 ½ cups of almond flour
- ¾ tsp. of baking powder
- ¼ tsp. of baking soda

- ¼ cup of unsweetened almond milk
- ¼ cup of almond butter
- ¼ cup of swerve
- 1 tbsp. of raw almonds, chopped
- 1 tsp. of raspberry extract

	Breakfast	Lunch	Dinner	Dessert
Sunday	Avocado stuffed with tuna	Cheeseburger calzone	Chicken and asparagus	Mini chocolate cakes
Monday	Tuna in cucumber	Cumin spiced beef wraps	Chicken Kiev	Poached eggs
Tuesday	Small keto pies	Portobello bun cheese burgers	Chicken pad thai	Ricotta lemon cheesecake
Wednesday	Keto wraps	BBQ pulled beef sando	Chicken parmesan	Wheat belly yoghurt
Thursday	Deviled eggs	Beef wellington	Chicken smothered in creamy onion	Eggs in a cup
Friday	Low-carb muffins with whey	Bone broth for BBQ	Chicken stuffed avocado	Vanilla bean cheesecake
Saturday	Spinach rolls	Mississippi chuck roast	Coconut curry chicken	Greek yoghurt

Week 2: Shopping List

- 12 eggs
- 4 oz. of (70/30) ground beef
- 4 tbsp. of BBQ sauce, sugar-free
- 4 bacon slices
- 1 ½ oz. of cheddar cheese
- 10 oz. of cream cheese
- 5 lbs. of chicken breasts
- 2 cups of diced cauliflower
- 2 tsp. of coconut curry
- 1 ½ cups of almond flour
- ½ cup of coconut flour
- ¼ cup of heavy cream
- ½ cup of fresh raspberries
- 5 egg yolks
- ¼ cup of butter
- 3 tsp. of powdered stevia
- 1 tsp. of baking powder
- 1 tsp. of vanilla extract, sugar-free
- ¼ cup of coconut oil

	Breakfast	Lunch	Dinner	Dessert
Sunday	Breakfast smoothie	Balsamic beef pot roast	Cordon bleu	Garlic spread
Monday	Low-carb breakfast balls	Cheeseburger calzone	Italian chicken and egg bake	Peanut butter cheesecake
Tuesday	Keto muffins with chicken	Vegetarian Keto burger	Italian chicken and cauliflower	Pumpkin pecan cake
Wednesday	Borecole with curry	Barbecue pulled chicken	Kung pao chicken	Chocolate cream
Thursday	Eggs on sour cream	Coconut curry chicken	Nacho chicken casserole	Butter pancakes
Friday	Low-carb bacon muffins	Ground beef bacon	Tikka masala chicken	Raspberry cookies
Saturday	Zucchini in yoghurt	BBQ and bacon cheeseburger	Pizza goodies BBQ meat lover's pizza	Vanilla mousse with chocolate

Week 3: Shopping list

- 2 tbsp. of pepper
- 2 cups of diced Cauliflower
- 14 eggs
- 14 oz. of brussel sprouts
- 2 lbs. of trimmed Asparagus
- 4 oz. of sliced smoked salmon
- ½ tbsp. of butter
- 2 tbsp. of fresh chives
- 2 tbsp. of prepared horseradish
- 3 avocados
- 10 oz. of pulled pork
- 5 beef tenderloin steaks
- 1 ½ cups of both green & purple cabbage
- 1 lb. of browned sausage
- ¼ tsp. of salt

- 1 tsp. ginger
- ¼ cup of protein powder
- 1 cup of pumpkin puree
- ¼ tsp. of cloves
- 1 tsp. of vanilla
- 1 ½ tsp. of cinnamon
- ¼ cup of butter, melted
- 2 tsp. of baking powder
- ⅓ cup of coconut flour
- ¾ cup of swerve
- 1 ½ cups of raw pecan

	Breakfast	Lunch	Dinner	Dessert
Sunday	Keto coconut bread	Salmon fishcakes	Beefy pizza	Sweet almond buns
Monday	Baked brussels sprouts with	Bistro steak salad	Chicken fried pork chops	Cocoa patties
Tuesday	Ketogenic protein muffins	Caprese salad	Parmesan crusted pork chops	Easy almond bars
Wednesday	Fried peppers cauliflowers	Egg salad stuffed avocado	Skillet sausage and cabbage	Pumpkin pie pancakes
Thursday	Eggs sauce	Thai pork salad	Squash and sausage casserole	Coconut brownies raspberry
Friday	Keto breakfast	Vegetarian club salad	Chili lime cod	Chocolate chip cookies
Saturday	Asparagus frittata	Cumin spiced beef wraps	Pan fried cod	Vanilla cream

Week 4: Shopping List

- 12 eggs
- 4 bacon slices
- 10 oz. of cream cheese
- 5 beef tenderloin steaks
- 1 ½ lbs. of salmon fillets
- 4 cups of almond flour
- 5 cups of dark chocolate, unsweetened
- 5 cups of raw cocoa powder
- 2 tsp. of powdered stevia
- 2 cups of almond milk, unsweetened
- 1 tsp. of baking powder
- 1 tsp. of baking soda
- ¾ cup of whipped cream
- ¾ cup of almond milk, unsweetened
- 4 egg whites
- 3 tsp. of powdered stevia
- 1 tsp. of cherry extract, sugar-free

	Breakfast	Lunch	Dinner	Dessert
Sunday	Scrambled eggs	Beef burritos	Grilled salmon	Peanut butter brownies
Monday	Bacon burger	Open-faced prosciutto	Sushi	Cherry pudding
Tuesday	Pesto scrambled	Keto cubano	Walnut crusted	Creamy raspberry cake
Wednesday	Keto cheese tacos	Keto monkey bread	One-pot shrimp alfredo	Strawberry chocolate fudge
Thursday	Keto donuts	Beef stew	Loaded tuna fish salad	Apple lemon pie
Friday	Chive and bacon omelet	Beef welly	Tuna tartare	Almond strawberry
Saturday	Keto waffles	Salmon fishcakes	Chipotle fish tacos	Chocolate chip Keto brownies

Chapter 13: Volume conversion tables

Table 1

1/16 teaspoon	A dash		
⅛ teaspoon or less	A pinch or 6 drops		.5 ml
¼ teaspoon	15 drops		1 ml
½ teaspoon	30 drops		2 ml
1 teaspoon	⅓ tablespoon	1/6 ounce	5 ml
3 teaspoons	1 tablespoon	½ ounce	14 grams
1 tablespoon	3 tablespoons	½ ounce	14 grams
2 tablespoons	⅛ cup	1 ounce	28 grams

4 tablespoons	¼ cup	2 ounce		56.7 grams
5 tablespoons plus 1 teaspoon	⅓ cup	2.6 ounces		75.6 grams
8 tablespoons	½ cup	4 ounces	¼ pound	113.4 grams
10 tablespoons plus 2 teaspoons	⅔ cup	5.2 ounces		158 ml
12 tablespoons	¾ cup	6 ounces	.375 pound	177ml
16 tablespoons	1 cup	8 ounces	½ pound	225 ml
32 tablespoons	2 cups	16 ounces	1 pound	450 ml

Table 2

Volume conversions: Normally used for liquids only

Customary Quantity	Metric Equivalent
1 teaspoon	5 ml
1 teaspoon or ½ fluid ounce	15 ml
1 fluid ounce or ⅛ cup	30 ml
¼ cup or 2 fluid ounces	60 ml
⅓ cup	80 ml
½ cup or 4 fluid ounces	120 ml
⅔ cup	160 ml
¾ cup or 6 fluid ounces	180 ml
1 cup or 8 fluid ounces of half a pint	240 ml
1 ½ cups or 12 fluid ounces	350 ml
2 cups or 1 pint or 16 fluid ounces	475 ml
3 cups or 1 ½ pints	700 ml
4 cups or 2 pints or 1 quart	950 ml

Conclusion

The Ketogenic Diet is perfect if you want to lose weight and improve your health. This book has explained all about the Ketogenic Diet and the balance of food. Not only will you lose weight, but your cholesterol will improve, your blood sugar and blood pressure will reduce and there's a wealth of other conditions/diseases you're at less risk of contracting when on the Ketogenic Diet. Thank you for downloading this book. It is my sincere hope that you will apply the acquired knowledge productively.

Made in the USA
Columbia, SC
26 August 2018